SUGAR RIDE

Cycling from Hanoi to Kuala Lumpur

YVONNE BLOMER

SUGAR RIDE

Cycling from Hanoi to Kuala Lumpur

Palimpsest Press / www.palimpsestpress.ca
1171 Eastlawn Ave. Windsor, Ontario. N8S 3J1

Book and cover design by Dawn Kresan. Bound and printed in Ontario, Canada. Edited by Carmine Starnino. Cover art by Regan Rasmussen.

Palimpsest Press would like to thank the Canada Council for the Arts, and the Ontario Arts Council for their support of our publishing program. We also acknowledge the assistance of the Government of Ontario through the Ontario Book Publishing Tax Credit.

 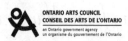

LIBRARY AND ARCHIVES CANADA CATALOGUING IN PUBLICATION

Blomer, Yvonne, author
    Sugar Ride: Cycling from Hanoi to Kuala Lumpur / Yvonne Blomer.

Issued in print and electronic formats.
ISBN 978-1-926794-39-6 (softcover)
ISBN 978-1-926794-46-4 (PDF)

1. Blomer, Yvonne–Travel–Southeast Asia. 2. Authors, Canadian Travel–Southeast Asia. 3. Cycling–Southeast Asia. 4. Southeast Asia–Description and travel. I. Title.

DS522.6.B56 2017   915.904'54   C2016-908120-6
                                              C2016-908121-4

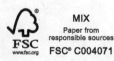

MIX
Paper from
responsible sources
FSC® C004071

for Rupert

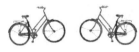

Hanoi, Vietnam, September 9, 1999 –
Kuala Lumpur, Malaysia, November 28, 1999

If one is to try to record one's life truthfully, one must aim at getting into the record of it something of the disorderly discontinuity which makes it so absurd, unpredictable, bearable.

—LEONARD WOOLF

It is by riding a bicycle that you learn the contours of a country best, since you have to sweat up the hills and coast down them. Thus you remember them as they actually are, while in a motor car only a high hill impresses you, and you have no such accurate remembrance of country you have driven through as you gain by riding a bicycle.

—ERNEST HEMINGWAY

Happy Halloween, Thailand, October 31

Will I ever catch up to him?

In his yellow shirt, he has pedaled so far ahead that he's almost out of sight. I want to stop for a rest. My hands, ass, legs, shoulders hurt. He is racing the wind or rain, has set a pace and is sticking to it, some overplayed Madonna song driving him.

"Rupert" I yell, knowing the futility of it.

Dropped in the middle of nowhere, I've forgotten the point of this exercise. I'm dizzy and light-headed. I need to eat. I stop, pull a PowerBar out of my bag and tear into it. It turns to paste in my mouth as I anxiously watch him become a spot on my glasses, a fleck of pollen in the air. *He who?* I drink water and quickly get going. *Where am I?* The little voice in my head becomes less and less comforting. *Who? Who?* I whisper to myself. *Apparition*, I think. *Ghost-husband.* He can just go straight to hell. Ride right off the edge of the world for all I care. Then a car full of guys revs alongside me.

"Hey," the driver says through his open window. "Where you go?"

I don't smile. Look ahead. *Keep pedaling.* Rupert has disappeared completely. *Who?* I ask myself again. *Who Rupert.*

"Hey. You speak English?"

I involuntarily nod, turn my head slowly, look the driver straight in the eyes.

"Where you going?" His friends leer, hang out the window. There are four of them. I point ahead and they laugh.

Rupert, Rupert, Rupert, Rupert, Rupert, I chant in my head. *Stop. Come back. Stop come back stop come back stop.* I look around. No small side roads, no small shops, nothing. I look at the driver again. Stupidly smile.

Sweat drips between my breasts, down my neck, down my back. My tongue is numb. I realize my blood sugars are very low. I can feel myself going under. I keep pedaling.

When I was ten years old, I learned that the reason I'd been getting up every hour in the night to pee, and the reason I was hungry all the time but also tired and thirsty and skinny and weedy looking was because I had diabetes. For two weeks I left my regular life of school and friends and silliness and stayed in the Edmonton General Hospital and learned how to be diabetic. The doctors and nurses taught me about calories and urine testing (later replaced by the more publicly acceptable blood testing) and I practiced giving injections to oranges while letting the nurses or my dad practice on me. I began to feel better once those first shots of pork-based insulin were jabbed into me. I learned how to measure and weigh food, eat regular meals, do injections and test urine so that by the time I returned home my parents and I were fully trained in how to live with diabetes.

In the hospital, a tall buxom nurse with upswept blond curls and bright red lips said two things to me. She said, KISS (Keep it Simple Sweetheart) and she told me never to use my diabetes as an excuse. As a child these two morsels entered my veins and filled the tissue around my organs and brain. They created a filter through which I looked at the world and through which I looked at myself.

"You should come with us," says the driver. "You stop."

I shake my head and keep pedaling. My vision is blurred. I feel drunk.

"Yeah, we need company," one in the back says, leaning out the window, waggling his hand at me.

I see a bus shelter, a yellow shirt inside. *Yellowshirtyellowshirtyellowshirt.*

A truck comes up behind the car, which now has to either pull over or speed up. The driver pulls behind me. I pedal as fast as I can, using the last few ounces of sugar in my body. Rupert sits in the bus shelter 500 metres ahead. The guys in the car see him, take a long look at me, all four of them, then pull back into traffic after the truck passes.

I wave to the truck driver, fly off my bike, yelling. Rupert stands up to catch me.

"Wait a minute sir/ you kind of hurt my feelings/ You see me as a sweet back-loaded puppet/ And you've got meal ticket taste" (Alanis Morissette, "Right Through You").

In two years in Japan I rarely told anyone I was diabetic. I didn't want the people, who were becoming friends, to think less of me. To consider me weak. Diabetes as a form of shame.

This is a condition that can be hidden from view. No one need know. Except… sometimes being both diabetic and a woman feels like double the weakness. Couldn't I just rely on myself for a change? Not fly, like some helpless maiden, into the puzzled arms of a man.

At twenty-one a friend gave me her classic Lady's Raleigh. At twenty-one I met Rupert at university. He was always clad in black leggings, army shorts overtop, a red plaid jacket and a faded black backpack with a silver helmet swinging from it. His straight blond-brown hair with long bangs swung over his blue eyes. Over six feet and lanky, he walked with a kind of high-altitude buoyancy. Partners, we measured each other's skulls in Archaeology lab.

Which love came first—Rupert or the bike? I remember beers in the Student Union Building and a ride home on his handlebars. Remember my first long solo ride on that Raleigh, up and down distant streets till my legs throbbed and ached. I rode that Raleigh until the cranks fell off and the bike could go no more. A Giant Hybrid replaced it. I married Rupert, who rode a Schwinn. We packed up our bikes and flew to Japan.

Our new employer, the Japanese Government, flew us First Class on Japan Airlines. We had been hired as Assistant Language Teachers in the JET Program. Newlyweds, we landed in Tokyo suddenly overwhelmed as Japanese words spilled from neon lights and off trains; they slid from menus and out of the mouths of fast-talking waiters.

Cycling to Hagi, bartering for soybeans, seeing Samurai and Noh plays, teaching and running English clubs, sampling fried oyster mushrooms, laughing under cherry blossoms with Japanese friends—we were too busy to notice how or when Japan had become home. After two years our time was coming to an end. We wanted to find a way to honour our lives in

Asia. We decided to embark on a three-month bicycle trip from Hanoi in Vietnam to Laos, Thailand, and finally fly home to Vancouver from Kuala Lumpur in Malaysia.

I'd gained a love of cycling with Rupert and I'd done a short bike tour in Thailand with a friend. It felt natural, exhilarating, daring even to travel the meandering thousands of kilometers from Hanoi west on bicycles. We would take our two perfect machines—give or take a dent, rust spot or creaky chain—on a long ride home.

Always on display, we learned to avoid public displays. Learned to walk through the shopping tunnels of Nōgata with our hands in our pockets. Elbows or shoulders touching. How this could translate as distance. Should we make love right here? Find a ramshackle guest house with a double bed? Better yet, instead of pulling plantains off the tree on the mountain in northern Thailand, pull me into the bushes. I am blind with conjunctivitis. Lay me down in the shade. I am weary with hills.

Hanoi, Vietnam, September 9

Groggy-eyed we enter this new world, our bikes boxed and teetering on an airport trolley. I squint beyond the parking lot to the mountains wrapped in shining emerald trees. Everything is wet with humidity and glowing. The bikes begin to slip.

"Yvonne!" Rupert yells, yanking me back into the hot day.

He slowly stops the trolley and I get my weight under and beside the bikes, hold them in place.

As I walk, my body pushed against the boxes and gear, I look around the small airport with its sprawling concrete parking area. I can hear the low hum of traffic in the distance. We spot shade at the back near the fence line and head there, passing a few cyclos lined up just beyond the airport entrance. The drivers watch us as we make our slow way. Beyond the fencing, I can make out the road, a few crumbling houses, trees and mountains that rise straight up. I take a deep breath, happy to be outside again, happy for the moisture in the air and the subtle scents of distant greenery, with an undertow of dusty dirt. We stop then Rupert and I carefully lift the boxes off the cart, place them on the ground, so the bikes lie on their sides, and open them. My heart leaps at the sight of my bicycle. Rupert and I lean into each other for a moment, then get busy lifting out each bike and lining up all the parts: wheels with flat tires, pedals in plastic bags, and semi-attached handlebars. We scrutinize both bikes for damage but they seem in good shape. The boxes are in ruin, but the bikes don't look bent or battered.

We barely speak as we assemble. Rupert helps me put my handle-bars on and then we flip my bike upside down so I can attach the wheels. He then does the same with his bike. We are sweating in minutes from the exertion and heat. I tie my hair off my face and push up my glasses. I would like to be one of those awesome women who are not shy about using a wrench or changing a flat tire. I am working on my skills here. Rupert, on the other hand, is a handy man. Not one of those guys to sit back and let other people get their hands dirty, he gets right in there. Sweat drips into my eyes and my glasses fog but I chant *you-can-do-it-you-can-do-it-youcandoit* in my head.

"Let me help," Rupert says, hovering.

"I can do it," I say, sweating as I pump tires.

The cyclo cabs, when I look up, are closer. The drivers watch in silence, look at each other every once in a while, then back at us, as if they can't believe we've come to Vietnam with bicycles. This is a country of bicycles. Maybe they think the bikes are some kind of foreign trick to get out of paying for a cab ride.

Hot and sticky, I dig in a pannier for a bandana to hold the stray hairs completely off my forehead and to catch the dripping sweat before bending over my tire with our small pump.

I stand to stretch and one of the cab drivers comes over to help. He takes the pump and begins to inflate the tire while his comrades look on. Another driver approaches to give the tire a squeeze, then shakes his head, lips pushed together teasingly, and gestures to keep pumping.

Rupert packs everything into his panniers and then mock-pouts at me: "Sure they can help." In his yellow cycling jersey, loose shorts over padded cycling shorts and runners, he is pink-faced and sweating. He towers over the drivers as he rolls past to entertain some kids on the far side of the fence, their faces pressed close, watching. They have bikes too, or so we think, and take up the task of bartering theirs for his.

While Rupert jokes around—all in gestures and nods—my cab driver finishes pumping. I bow a thanks, screw the valve tight, clumsily fit my awkward panniers to my bike, then run inside to change into my cycling shorts and buy water.

We should have thought of buying water first, because the airport, by this time, is shut down. I use the toilet. The tap water is not drinkable so from a small kiosk I buy two 250ml bottles of water with the few American dollars I have in my pocket. The money exchange is closed, so we have nothing. We have no idea how long it will take to ride to Hanoi or if we'll be able to find more drinkable water. It's about thirty-six degrees Celsius.

Back outside, I see Rupert, in playful gestures challenging one of the kids to follow us. They all laugh then ride off on one bicycle. We'd thought they each had their own, but in fact they all share one: three gangly passengers and one cyclist. Suddenly our loads look comical, a luxury of travel clothes and knick-knacks in a country where the bicycle truly is a vehicle of transport, play and work.

We are about thirty kilometres from Hanoi, in the Red River Valley. We have been living in Japan for the past two years. Adept at bowing our thanks. Adept at catching the attention of those around us. I walk toward Rupert, psyching myself up to ride.

"I should test my blood," I say, preventing Rupert from pushing off toward the highway. "4.2. A little low. Do you want some PowerBar?"

"Not really," he says as he takes a hearty bite. We roll toward the exit, wait, then signal left, enter the bike-buffalo-moped traffic heading for the city.

As we crested the overpass that crossed the Red River, I was split in two. My body on the weighted wobble of my bike. Sweat running down my back, down my shorts and into my socks. My eyes and sense of smell, my ears: the green, the red dirt and ochre water, the swarms of people, scents of buffalo, rotting pig, garlic cooking, diesel fuel, dust in my nose. My head full of the honk and hum of life. I wanted to yell out to Rupert, to nudge him with my elbow and say "Look look look." He focused on the narrow pathway, mosaic of traffic, the climb, his body on bike. I saw how his long limbs, white skin, distracted everyone he passed. I was humming behind him. Humming still. Caught, still, on that overpass in that throng of bodies and beauty.

In the dark theater, before the puppets enter the stage, it is silent but for the sound of water tickling itself. The stage is a red roofed temple-like building called a *dinh* and the sets float on a shallow pool of water. The scene: a house with an open balcony in the foreground of the temple. A little boy puppet floats across the water to introduce the story. We can't see the puppeteers at all. They stand in the water behind a bamboo screen holding the puppets' long poles. From the boy's introduction, one story drifts into the next as brightly costumed puppets glide on and off stage. Stories of rural life in Vietnam show fishermen with their mini nets dipping and dipping as if into a river, followed by women planting rice hand over hand into wet fields, and water buffalo snorting and plodding their way across a country hemmed in by fuzzy green mountains. We move from daily life to the smoke and rapid-fire of fighting until the puppets tire of reliving the war. The scene ends with a fisherman resting under a banyan tree. The music squeaks and brays in the timbre of wooden flutes and tin drums. I hear the wind, bird song, shuffling feet, whining wheels, the heft of labour, and the rub of worn tires on gravel in the voice of this music. I have a sense of what lies ahead before I've seen the country itself. The road will point the way ahead, to villages, temples, people's house fronts, the graves of men who died in war and their children's children yelling after us. These children are also parents, farmers, shop keepers, labourers and keepers of their country's uncertain future and its difficult past.

I am writing on the threshold. Of place and history. Of dissonance and longing. Between this time and that one. I am in my twenties and newly married. I am in my forties with a ten year old and a long marriage. I am stretching my fingers to touch on multiple perceptions. Composite. Story, like time, is flexible and not always chronological. How our perception of what we experience can change with knowledge. My first instinct, pre-You Tube and Google, was less-informed but still accurate.

On the water-stage everything is mirror: flexible, changeable, fickle before the audience's eye.

After the puppets we walk back to our hotel along Hoan Kiem Lake, through the centre of the city. We pass three cyclo drivers who follow us with their eyes. Then I sense their attention jump to a little girl, approaching.

"Please," she holds her hand out for money. Seconds later, her grandmother grabs her begging hands and pulls her away, bowing at us as she marches the child off.

One of the cyclo drivers coasts over, "We are too proud, we will not allow our children to beg. You will see begging in the South, but not here, not in the North."

Rupert and I nod to the driver, and look back to watch the grandmother and child. "Wherever we go, we'll always stand out," I say, looking up at him as we continue.

"I wonder if he's right," Rupert muses. "I wonder if we won't see much begging up here, but will once we enter the Demilitarized Zone."

Rupert's thoughts trail off as we continue along the lake, noting the bridge that crosses over to the Ngoc Son Temple and the few people going home or to work, to hotels or a late night café. Our guest house is in the old quarter where every street is named after the trade and merchants on that street. We pass Woven Basket Street where women hunch over large weaving mats and Tin Street where merchants pound tin pots and bins into the wee hours of the night. In our room, I restlessly toss beside my heavy-sleeping husband and imagine the road ahead.

At the puppet theatre I watched a turtle push a temple up from under the water. Then the turtle had something in its mouth. Then smoke filled the water and the temple sank. What was the turtle holding in its mouth? What were the men doing in their boats rowing toward and away, toward and away from the turtle?

Years later, I read about the rare Yangtze giant softshell turtle. Only four remained in existence until January of 2016 when the Hoan Kiem Lake turtle is believed to have died. It was over one-hundred years old. In Vietnamese folklore that very turtle was thought to be the Golden Turtle God who rescued the country many times. In the stories, a fisherman pulled a sword out of the lake and gave it to a lord who used it to fight for Vietnam's independence from China in the fifteenth-century. The boats in the puppet theatre must have been the fisherman and the lord. The lord became emperor and when he returned to the lake, the Golden Turtle poked his head up and asked for the sword to be returned. The story is ancient, as was the turtle, but carries within it the many battles Vietnam has fought for independence, including the more recent Vietnam War.

Fragments from the road

Hot and restless in a dark room with yellow walls and translucent curtains, my heel hooked on the bottom tube of my Giant. My husband breathing the breath of the sleeping. Hanoi.

Standing half-naked, my hair fizzed with shampoo in an irrigation pond. Thailand.

IV tube in my wrist, fluids and anti-nausea drugs drip into my sleeping body. Rupert in a chair, reading. He could look up to the window, to the rich green slope of the Cameron Highlands' tea bushes. I turn, open my eyes. Malaysia.

Born in Zimbabwe (Rhodesia), I was an infant when my parents immigrated to Canada. From one colony to the other. From Africa and years of coloniza-tion to Canada and its horrors of residential schools and missing women. Born to British parents who were drawn to the heat and adventure, drawn to the privilege even if they didn't see it. Even if they are good people. Even if I am colour blind. Even if I want to reach out a hand, the hand is white and it carries all the baggage of colour. Will we ever free ourselves of this colour-trap? Free ourselves of our need to judge and rank?

Riding unpaved highway toward Pho Len, Vietnam, September 13

Today Vietnam will begin to repave its entire national highway. I stand on pedals to coast for a while over loose gravel, dodge the bigger rocks and smile at the men and women moving broken asphalt in baskets on their heads or tied to bikes. I tuck my nose into my shirt to avoid dust and the smell of tar as I pedal hard to stay close to Rupert. He rides standing. I sit and push, stand and coast, though the word "coast" sounds smooth. To bump along, to joint and muscle grind. The bike is heavy, packed to the gills with panniers and we are still negotiating the fine-tuning of balance with all the weight.

That weight is made up of two sets of cycling clothes each, one set of long pants and two t-shirts for regular wear, a sarong which will be blanket, skirt, dress and beach towel, a jar of peanut butter imported into and brought from Japan, and PowerBars my sister brought from Canada. Divided between our bags we have extra pen needles, cartridges of two kinds of insulin, slow-acting which is absorbed over the day and gives a basal dose and fast-acting absorbed with meals to give a bolus, test strips, and alcohol swabs. If one of us loses everything, I'll still have enough drugs to survive. We also have a medical kit which includes suture tapes and all manner of antiseptics, rehydration salts in case something we eat or the heat wears our bodies down. Each day at six p.m. sharp, we take an anti-malarial drug that makes us feel queasy for hours after. Each day I administer four injections of insulin, one of slow-acting to give a buffer of insulin and one for each meal of fast-acting to cover meals. In my handlebar bag I carry my blood tester and insulin pen kit with needles and test strips for the day, a camera, purse with the our day's money, sun screen and a photocopied map.

I also pack copy of *Geist* magazine, a novel (*Smilla's Sense of Snow* that I will read and discard, pick up a John Grisham in its place somewhere along the way), a just-begun journal, an atlas of Thailand in Thai, photocopied pages from out of date *Lonely Planet* books from the few English books in a Kitakyushu language school, for Vietnam, Laos, Thailand and Malaysia, toiletries that include lip cream, toothbrush and paste, face cream and a brush, a couple of handkerchiefs to tie my hair back, a small bag of Canada pins and tattoos, camera and film, and a letter in Vietnamese from a Vietnamese-American friend in Japan who had her dad translate explaining all the drugs we carry. Rupert has a battered copy of the Bible from the "English Library" I created and housed in our apartment. Not because he's religious, but because he's always wanted to read it cover to cover, for the stories and mythologies that pervade the Western world.

"I need a break." I holler to be heard over the smashing of road and raking of gravel. We pull over, drink water, watch the people around us endlessly dig and fill and carry. Fleetingly I wish they were knee-deep in water, like the puppets of a few days ago.

"Man!" Rupert says, shaking his head as he watches the cloud of churned-up road coat us and all the workers.

We have been travelling at a snail's pace today because of the road surface. We are dust-coated and weary already.

"OK, let's keep going," I sigh, while munching on a piece of dried mango. Rupert drains his bottle, pulls the next one off the top of his pannier, just shoved under the rain cover, and away we go.

In Victoria these days the bicycle is a commuter vehicle. It is how parents get kids to school, how musicians carry their cellos and kayakers their boats. There are improbable options in trailers—cargo bikes, bikes with engines. In

Southeast Asia the bike seemed equivalent to the labouring horse, ideal for a labouring people. I felt a kinship to them on that gravel road, spewing dust back at myself. Every mile of the highway an open slash being stitched closed again, bucket by bucket, loaded bike by loaded bike. This too must have changed by now, by now big trucks and the highway repaved again.

Pied Piper, Vietnam, September 12

Late-morning we stop near the entrance to a train station. Rupert walks up to the building to find a toilet and garbage can. I wait with the bikes and watch a row of children follow him: "Hello!," "What's your name?," "Where you from?," "Where are you going?" These questions are followed by more detailed questions in Vietnamese. He answers as he goes, then asks an adult for a toilet. The man points back to the road and says something sharp, a reprimand perhaps, to the kids.

"He's pointing to that tree," I suggest. I can see no other options.

Rupert, the Pied Piper, looks behind him. The kids lean against a wall in the shade to watch, giggles erupting up and down the line of them. He shrugs and heads for the tree.

Two girls, one in pink shorts and matching shirt, the other in soccer shorts and a striped t-shirt, tiptoe quickly after him. They follow him down the drive, stretching their necks to see but not be seen. Then, giggling, run back to their cohort to send the next spy.

Rupert is unfazed by this. I can see from the look on his face that he is contemplating some mischief. I raise my eyebrows at him. He could chase the kids, swoop one up playfully in his arms. Then again, he is a big white guy and what he and I know to be friendly could be mistaken.

As Rupert swings his leg over his bike, I notice that the heat is slowing him down too; even the smallest leg-swing is an effort.

Rupert is cautious and sensible in how he lives, how he enters the world, how he approaches things. But he also has a wicked sense of humour. In Japan he visited elementary schools in our area for months. At each one he taught the kids how to do self-introductions by doing his own. As a Brad Pitt look-alike (to the Japanese, that is), with towering height, shorn blonde hair and a mischievous smile, he'd tell the kids stories: "Hello. My name is Rupert Gadd. I have two brothers. I am married. I live in an igloo in Canada. I ride a bicycle to work. My younger brother is a grizzly bear wrestler." He would recount the details of his life with photographs or hand-drawn pictures. The students would have to guess what parts of his biography were true, what parts false. Sometimes the false stories were so subtle, the true ones accompanied by hand-drawn pictures to throw the kids off.

By noon we are hungry for lunch, so pull off the highway into a clearing of trees, lean our bikes against a log and lean against them. Standing feels good at this point, though the muscles tighten. Wherever we stop, a crowd gathers and this time is no exception. The custom in Vietnam is silence during meals, so we are left to our snack while people stand around and watch. The group starts, as it always does, with a few children. Then, since we seem to be settling in for a bit, one child runs off and returns with a few adults who are slowly joined by others from nearby farms and houses. Rupert and I lean into our bikes, chewing, whispering to each other in growing wonder at our own novelty. I pull out the dried mango and offer it around but no one accepts. I say, "We come from Hanoi," pointing back. "We are going to Phu Ly," pointing forward, conscious of my accent and pronunciation. Everyone laughs. I try the "small talk" section of our Vietnamese phrase book—"Lovely day isn't it". This meets with rigorous head-nodding approval. A child comes forward holding her grandmother's hand. A young man approaches. He speaks in halting English and takes a piece of the offered fruit. The crowd stops speaking to watch him eat. A few minutes later, everyone begins to talk again. Then, a woman, maybe their mom, in a long cotton shirt and loose pants, is pushed forward by some kids; she reaches up and touches my hair, says something back to the kids. Another woman comes forward and pats me on the head. No one touches Rupert. They just stand near him and smile. Rupert and the young man chat for a bit, but once he wanders off, everyone begins to disperse.

It was uncommon to see tourists in the northern parts of Vietnam, especially tourists on bicycles. We were the anomalies. We the others. Everything has shifted since then. Opened to the world market, Vietnam is more developed. It has expanded to high-rises, shrunk from farms and country roads.

Our first long day is gruelling, the heat debilitating. My insulin is also sensitive to the heat, so as we pull over by a small road-side stand and lean our bikes on a tree. Rupert grabs our change wallet from my handlebar bag and I dig in my pannier to check the cold water-bottle next to my spare insulin.

"Are there frozen bottles in the cooler?" I ask as he moves bottles to get to the very back and pulls out two solid bottles. These will keep my insulin, buried in the bottom of the panniers, cold. Rupert also gets a coke and a bag of chips.

I have packed the insulin in one pannier and in the other cold-sensitive test strips in Ziploc bags, hundreds of small needles, like nibs for a pen that screw onto a pen-cartridge. I dial the amount I need and inject. I've divided the needles into four small bags. With four or five injections a day over three months this adds up to four hundred and sixty. However, I have packed over five hundred just in case I need more plus vials of Regular (fast acting) and NPH (slow acting) each of which contains 10ml or 100 units. I take 25 units of NPH a day and 15 units of Regular, but the dose goes up and down depending on food and exercise. In order to know how much insulin to take, I test my blood three to five times a day. This requires three hundred and seventy test strips, lancets, which are tiny sharp-pointed blood testing blades, and alcohol swabs. Basically, half of one pannier and a third of one of Rupert's contains drugs or drug paraphernalia. In my handlebar bag I carry my insulin kit, which is a small zippered pouch with the two pens with Regular and NPH insulin, blood testing machine and spare strips, lancets and alcohol strips for daily use. I don't need to dig into all the spare things until the end of the day, when I replace what I used.

Rupert sat back in the shade of that roadside stand and downed his Coke. Our first day out of Hanoi and already the heat was a tyranny even he couldn't escape. Over the coming months he would acclimatize to the heat, or suffer stomach woes. He would also revel in six dollar guest rooms, focus on the distance between towns and food. The vagaries of my health were always present

in his mind just as my ability to handle the demands of my body was a given between us, steady as road beneath and sun above. His body too, though, needed rest, food, and water every hour. He felt better when he followed the more vocal needs of my diabetic body.

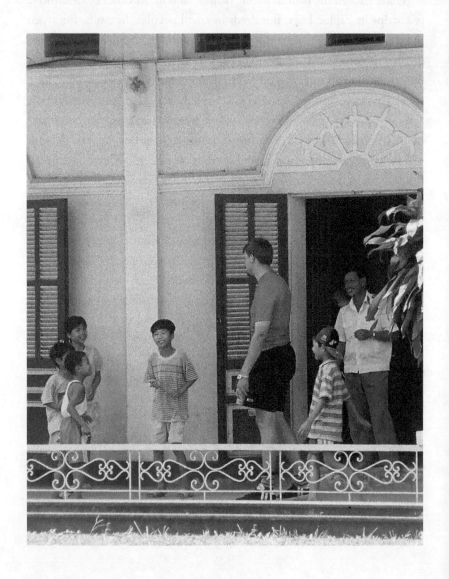

Naklang Midnight Resort, Thailand, October 12

A white Toyota pickup stops outside our small tile-roofed bungalow. I pull on my rayon slacks, drop my towel on the bed and quickly finger-comb my hair before stepping outside. "Hey," I say to the man getting out of his truck.

"Hi," he smiles back. "Can I drive you to town for dinner? I am the owner of this hotel. We are outside of town a little."

"Oh!" I am in a half-bow when Rupert comes out behind me.

"That would be great," he says and gives a little bow. I run back in to grab the back pack, shove in my insulin kit and tuck my money belt under my waistband. We pile into the truck, me in the middle.

At the restaurant our new friend tells us he has already eaten dinner but is happy to have a beer with us while we wait for our food and eat. He speaks a little English, with Thai words interrupting the flow. He looks to be in his early-thirties and has two children. He and his wife bought the guesthouse a year ago. The Thai words that interrupt his English start sounding strangely familiar when he says, "Is it samui, uh, cold in Canada?"

While Rupert answers, my mind gets stuck mulling over his words. *Samui? Did he say samui? Cold in Thai sounds a lot like cold in Japanese.* Then it happens again.

"You are very takai, tall," he says to Rupert.

"Can you speak Japanese?" I ask.

He smiles and tells us he lived there, on and off, teaching Thai kick-boxing. He also visited as a tourist, which I find incredible. The average Thai could never afford to travel to Japan. He must have earned good money teaching Kick boxing. We switch to Japanese, interjecting a few English words.

"Japanese people were very good to me," he says, "so I wanted to be good to you, to help you while you are in Thailand."

Images linger—Number 10 Guest House at Naklang Midnight Resort. Bikes under the low awning. Red tin roof. Low door. Rupert in a rattan chair, Chang beer in hand.

Later in Laos we met a young Japanese cyclist riding in flip flops, a near empty backpack bungeed to the back of his gorgeous fat-tired mountain bike. We sat in the shade with him and chatted in Japanese. He was shy with us but also delighted that we could speak Japanese. He didn't have any water, so I gave him one of my full bottles. We showed him the way to the Friendship Bridge so he could cross into Thailand. We all bowed when we parted ways. We were Canadian once removed; in some ways, we had become Asian.

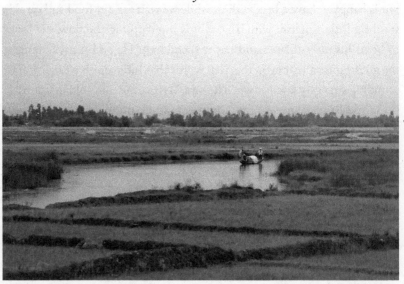

"Is that a restaurant?" Rupert points to what looks like a living room with plastic tables and chairs. We walk past noting three women inside, cross the street, walk back, cross again. As we enter, our heads automatically bob in bows. The eldest woman points to a table. We sit and I dig our phrasebook out of my fanny-pack.

"Toi an chay," I try, adding accents where they are marked while Rupert nods. "*I am vegetarian.* There, so, what shall we have?" I look at Rupert.

Without menus we use the food section of the phrase book and try to find something simple. After a few attempts, we show our waitress the Vietnamese for "noodles and vegetables." She nods then looks at Rupert.

"Chan nem" he says, holding the book out and pointing. The woman smiles and walks off. "Huh, that wasn't so bad."

The youngest woman—I begin to think of them as sisters—grabs some cash from the register, hops on a bike and rides off down the street. My first thought is that the town is bigger than we realize. Has she popped out to buy the spring rolls Rupert just ordered?

"Maybe they're out of tofu," Rupert suggests. We are hungry but have little confidence in what we've ordered. I am beginning to suspect that spring rolls and tofu are rare commodities, as rare here in small town Vietnam as tofu once was in small town Alberta or Ontario back home. The younger sister returns a few minutes later carrying a plastic bag with something lumpy and white inside. Rupert and I nod sagely to each other and relax.

"Phong tam?" I try, standing to find the toilet. The woman with long hair who I think of as the eldest, points me down the hall. The restaurant consists of a front area, where we are sitting, and a long corridor down the centre. The kitchen is on my left as I pass to turn right into the toilet. After washing my hands, I take out my insulin kit, test my blood sugars and inject four units of fast-acting Regular insulin to cover dinner. On my way back to the table, I notice an elderly woman—the mother?—bleeding a chicken in the kitchen. For a moment I stand and watch its blood drip into a bowl before walking back to Rupert.

"What?" he asks.

"It looks like the mother is the chef and she's bleeding a chicken. Did anyone else order food, do you think?" We look around. The place is empty. "Maybe they're killing their best chicken for us," I suggest, sweat gathering at the back of my neck and in my armpits. "What are we going to do?"

Being a hard core vegetarian is one of the potentially most difficult aspects of travelling in a foreign country, while also trying to honour the lives and respecting the customs of the people. I can't possibly eat the chicken in our noodle soup. I look up at Rupert, but he just shrugs.

We wait until eldest sister brings the soup, and indeed chunks of fresh chicken float in the liquid along with a few greens, garlic and plenty of noodles. I hold my head in my hands, whisper, "Can I just eat it?"

"No," Rupert says.

Phrase book in hand, I put my finger over "vegetarian" for eldest sister to see.

"Ahhhhh" she exclaims, followed by a stream of what I take to be apologies, followed by giggles and several embarrassed bows. Rupert says, no problem, he will eat both bowls of chicken noodles. A moment later, a bowl of noodles cooked in water arrives at the table. No greens, no tofu, nothing. Middle sister drops a plate of roadside veg on our table. I bow my thanks and dig in.

A moment later, Rupert's "spring rolls" are dropped in front of him. In fact, we have no idea what the youngest sister has placed before him. I look; he pokes with a chopstick.

"Lard," I offer.

Between us, on a white plate, sit five large, odd-shaped cubes of grey-God-knows-what. Rupert cuts a piece off and nibbles. "Hmmm."

I pick up a piece and smell it, then put it down. "Maybe different areas have different words for different foods," I offer. "Maybe spring rolls are tourist food. Maybe this is a lump of, of, really hard tofu."

Rupert scowls, deeply disappointed. He chopsticks his noodle soups.

Expectation and experience collide, or that frown when what you just put in your mouth tasted of sewer water and not the salted spicy spring roll you were expecting. How to reconcile what your body wants with what is available? I wonder if cultural differences can sometimes be reduced to food. My doctor who was moving to Saudi Arabia asked me, a couple of years after we returned from Japan, what to take. Favourite foods, I said. Take snacks. Junk food. Take what you crave.

We begin to relax, order second beers, when eldest sister comes to sit at the next table. She reaches out for the phrase book and flips through it.

"Canada," I say pointing at Rupert, then myself. We communicate in gestures, grunts and nods. Eldest sister asks where we are going. We point at the road—"Hanoi," we say, then point ahead—"Hue." We mime bicycle riding.

Middle sister joins us and takes the book. She sits next to me so eldest sister pulls up her chair on the other side. At first, they don't get too close to Rupert. They want to know how old we are, but don't believe it when I say twenty-eight.

"No, no, no," eldest sister says, while middle sister giggles. "Twenty-two."

Youngest sister joins us, sitting right next to Rupert and blinking prettily at him. He raises his eyebrows to me: "I think this is a brothel."

"Don't be silly, it's a family-owned business."

After an hour or so, hunched over in discussion and gestures, we notice the restaurant filling up. An elderly man comes forward looking for staff, but moves away from us and sits. Eldest sister gets him a beer and then comes back. A few other men straggle in off the street, dressed in jeans or overalls like car mechanics or construction workers. They settle down to play cards and chat, keeping an eye on our mingling.

"Married?" asks youngest sister.

We both nod in response.

"Children?"

I shake my head.

"Tsk, tsk," seems to be the reply. The sisters' pursed lips and sucked-in cheeks say it all.

In Japan, as in Asia, we were visible minorities. Sometimes this was merely an annoyance. A groceries- examined-at-the-check-out-and-photos-taken-on-the-train-kind-of-annoyance. Sometimes it was a delight. Lonely travellers in a quiet city, curious girls or women, conversation and a sense of connection. Where would you rather be? In the last class of my Anthropology degree one of my profs said to the students, "I hope you all go out into the world and place yourselves in situations where you know nothing, and can learn much."

In our room that night I sit on my cot alone with my thoughts, listening to Rupert breathe deeply in sleep. The distant traffic hums outside the window. While I wait to take my bedtime slow-acting injection I write in my journal. My eyes fall to the shape of our bikes against the wall as I replay our earlier conversation on the bridge over the Day River. We stood in the middle to gain a view of the orange-streaked sky. The bridge seemed to separate the rough part of town from the downright danger-ous part. We caught the scent of pot and could see discarded needles and other drug paraphernalia along the edge of the river.

"Mountains," I said, pointing to the right, down the length of the val-ley ahead. "Is that our path tomorrow?"

We stood side by side in silence watching the sunset, and then Rupert said, "This is one of those moments."

"What do you mean?"

"If life is about the small moments you remember forever, maybe this is one of them."

"It's only our first day," I said, leaning my back into his shoulder. "Maybe there will be a million moments like this."

"We don't know what's in front of us. Only right now." Rupert said.

"I wonder what's ahead. What we'll find on the road ahead. If we'll be ok. If we'll make it." I paused and then said, "We will make it."

Rupert put his arms around me, then seeing a small group of men approaching, he took my hand and drew me back toward the main road to find some dinner.

In our darkened room, I run my fingers over our map to flatten the creases. The main road snakes and winds left and right, up and down the length of the country. We have no idea where the road will take us—into the mountains or along the coast or both. I tuck the map into my journal, take my injection and turn off the lamp hopeful of sleep and a smooth road.

Where were we going? This question feels larger than the trip, feels expansive as life. What am I rooting around for? How did a story about the simple immediacy of action and adventure become something deeper? Who were we anyway? I look at my husband tonight, listen to our conversations and wonder what we have talked about all these years but housework, travel plans, career choices. With so much behind us, looking at him now pulls me into two parallel times and places. How what I thought then was a water buffalo sleeping in the shade I know now is a pile of coconut husks that had fallen, mounded just so.

To Chai Nat, 200 km from Bangkok, Thailand, October 20

Rupert slides up beside me on his bike, "Give me some sugar, baby," he says.

I blow him a raspberry and he pries my hand from the handlebars and kisses my knuckles, careful not to throw me off balance, then falls back to his place in the wide shoulder.

If I listen hard I can hear, beyond traffic and the hum of bike on asphalt, birds, dogs, children laughing. Sounds that place me exactly where I am on the road. I remember the tranquil silence of Laos, the moments of silence when there were no cars and serenity sank into me. Here, so close to Bangkok, there is noise but also moments when the traffic thins and the world is held in the silence of my spinning wheels. I re-enter my body, feel my leg muscles as they spin, my numb right toe, the crick in my right knee and the aching hum in my buttocks. When traffic picks up again, I let my thoughts wander off. Often I revisit movies and today, because we are getting close to a city, perhaps, or because my health is often on my mind, I think of *Steel Magnolias.*

Dolly Parton's sing-song advice rings in my head: add ice cream to a desert to cut the sugar, wear shoes three sizes too large because they are comfortable. I also love Parton's weird sayings such as "Busier than a one armed paper hanger," and "I'd rather walk on my lips than criticize anybody." I love the movie's cluster of female friends, something I had a taste of in Japan but never before. Too set on doing my own thing, I often seemed to alienate friends. In the movie, all the women are in-tune with each other. Maybe I've been with this man as my sole companion for too long, I think. Maybe I'm ready to hang with some women for an afternoon. Ready for a day that is not about sugar, whether keeping blood sugars in control or kissing the big lug.

I was a teenager when I watched *Steel Magnolias*, a movie about a group of women who support the Sally Fields character whose daughter, played by Julia Roberts, struggles with Type 1 diabetes, a diabetes that was alien to me. How could she die from it? What did the people who made the movie know that I didn't? I was aware and afraid of the possibilities such as blindness, loss of circulation, foot amputations and kidney disease. I understood the damage that was potentially going on in my body all the time due to the ups and downs that puberty, changes in hormone levels, activity and food were making in my body, but I didn't believe I had a life-threatening illness. The possibilities were on my radar, but every blood test came back normal; sometimes my sugars were good and sometimes bad. My yearly eye test results came back with no signs of diabetic retinopathy or small bumps in the tiny vessels of the eye. No problems with my kidneys. Good cholesterol was high, bad was low. There was more to the story, I felt, in *Steel Magnolias*, though I did harbour doubts about having children and my health certainly wasn't always perfect. If diabetes was causing damage to my body, it was happening very slowly.

On my bike all these weeks, though, I was aware of my health in very specific terms. I felt sluggish and wired. My eyes were puffy and some days my ankles were too. Could something be going on that I wasn't aware of? I should have collapsed into bed after every exhausting, hot day's ride, but I didn't. I sat up awake, suffering some version of FoMo…hoping we'd not missed anything that day.

Rupert pedals up beside me, breaking my reverie. "You okay?" he asks.

"Just thinking about a movie."

"What movie?"

"*Steel Magnolias*."

"Pink is my signature colour," he says in a mock-Southern accent.

I wag my head and imitate Julia Roberts' accent: "I'd rather have thirty minutes of wonderful than a lifetime of nothing special." As Shelby, Roberts decides to have a child against doctor's wishes. Her kidneys fail due to diabetes' complications and she dies. Chances are, in the early 1980s, she was on pork-based insulin and testing only her urine. She may have had kidney trouble before getting pregnant, as was more common then.

"Dolly Parton." Rupert says, wiggling his eyebrows, which wiggle his helmet.

"Yes, and Daryl Hannah."

We ride on, in silence. I fall back, coast in Rupert's slipstream. I remember that the men in the movie are secondary—they hardly matter—and the friendship between the five women centres around a beauty salon. On her wedding day, after Julia Robert's character has her hair done, her sugars drop. At first she is chatty, silly and excited, then she goes quiet, sweating. The sounds around her become distant and hollow, cave-like. She yells at her mother and everyone knows right away what is going on. Because her sugar levels are low, she doesn't know what she needs. She resists juice and candies. She just wants her purse, something from her purse, which she hasn't brought. As she is recovering, her mother says the doctors have told Shelby children aren't possible.

I return to my bike. A shiver of goosebumps runs up my arms, despite the fact that the temperature is thirty-eight degrees. I talk to myself, not having decided about kids yet. Then I look around, stand on pedals and pedal fast to catch up to Rupert. I've fallen back into thoughts, and he's kept going.

I re-watched Steel Magnolias *recently. The things I found strange as a teen—such as Julia Roberts never giving herself an injection and appearing so healthy —still niggle. Her low blood sugar reaction is awesomely done. As I watched, Rupert made a cheeky comment, in Shelby's southern accent: "But I never have lows like that!" I gave him a withering look. "Remember those mornings I couldn't wake you and then you'd be mad because your mouth tasted of yogurt drink?"*

Harrumph.

A friend says Steel Magnolias *made her fear diabetes. Another friend wondered if having an illness from a young age separates you, which may be why I'm so drawn to the friendship of those women. As I watched the movie again, I felt connected to the mother, for to be connected to Shelby is to contend with my own death. If I were a character in the movie, I'd be dead. After I watched, I did some research. Diabetes is the most common cause of kidney failure and yet as a typical teen, I did feel invincible. I was more aware of my own mortality because of the diabetes but I also believed I was as close to invincible as my peers. Now in my forties, I have to revisit the eye specialist so he can take a closer look at my right eye. A physio called my beginning-to-freeze left arm "diabetic frozen shoulder" to which I baulked. "A circulation issue," he repeated, looking down his nose at me. "Due to diabetes."*

Guest House, South of Ha Tinh, Vietnam, September 17

We round a corner going uphill and spot a sign for the Nha Nghi Mui Bao Guest House. I slow to let Rupert pull up beside me. "Shall we stop here?"

"Yes."

Never has a decision been so easy. We have gone close to eighty kilometers and are nearly at the base of the Ngang Pass. It will be so much nicer to do it in the morning, after a rest, and there may not be another guest house for hours.

From the road, it doesn't look like much. We roll then drag and heave our bikes down a set of stairs. The back looks quite lovely, with a row of simple attached suites and an ocean view.

"I wonder if there is a reception area at the front, near the café." Just as Rupert turns to go look, a woman and two men appear.

"Bao nhieu mo idem?" I ask.

We think the woman says 120,000 dong. I nod, and we continue toward the five rooms lined along the back of the building. She opens one door after the other until I choose one in the middle. Clean, it has the usual two beds, fan, cold shower and squat toilet. Rupert nods his assent; we pay and unload the bikes.

As I pull my paniers off and carry them inside, the woman hovers, watching me dump each item in the room. She gestures at my bike, wanting to ride it. I lower the seat and she rides up and down the boardwalk in front of the rooms, talking and gesturing to her male companions.

"Keep your hands on the handlebars," I say, mimicking a holding position. She grabs the handlebars before toppling. We laugh and she gets off and leans the bike against the outside wall.

She follows me into the room and as I get out my stuff-sack of toiletries, she sits on the bed. Each item fascinates her. She picks things up, holds them out to me, points to herself and gestures keeping it. I shake my head each time.

"We need that for sunburn. No, that is my lip cream." I point to my lips. "How will I brush my hair?" We continue in this vein until finally I dig in my bag and find a pink handkerchief, one of the many farewell handkerchiefs I was given in Japan. I have brought four to tie my hair back under my helmet, but I haven't used the pretty pink one. I hand it to her. She holds it to her chest, bowing and smiling as she leaves the room. It would have made more sense, I think, as I watch her go, to bring more of that kind of thing. The Japanese handkerchiefs are so delicate and beautiful and useful in this heat. I shove the Canada pins and tattoos into the bottom of my pack.

We don swim suits instead of diving into the cold shower. We know there are probably jelly fish in the water, but the beach looks sandy and the water inviting and we can't resist an ocean swim. Afterward, we walk to the front of the building to the café for a dinner of fried rice. Hungry, I take the first mouthful, dig into the second while chewing, then freeze mid-chew.

"This tastes funny."

Rupert nods, noncommittally.

"Does yours taste funny?"

"How do you mean?"

"Are you being difficult? It tastes greasy. My mouth feels coated in thick grease. Maybe it wasn't cooked in oil."

After quietly chewing on his own rice for a moment, he says, "I think it's been cooked in lard. There aren't a lot of options here. Maybe you have to eat it."

Suddenly I feel the truth of being off the highway with no town in sight. We are miles from anything remotely civilized, like a grocery store.

Even to those with mopeds and trucks, the nearest town is 100km away. Not that far, but remote for my particular vegetarian-diabetic needs.

I nod, drink water, eat another mouthful. When the waiter comes over, I order beer. *Chew, chew, chew, swallow* echoes the mantra. I've not had pig-fat in my mouth since I was twelve years old. I worry about my stomach, but eat the whole serving for the low blood sugars I've been battling all day. Rupert is right, I have limited options.

As we approached the Ngang Pass I struggled to keep my blood sugars up. We would face my worst low. We were edgy. We were constantly being saved by the people we met, people who wanted nothing from us but friendship. It heartened us. In the belly of my belly it made me laugh: some of the conversations, some of the roads, the rocks and rain made me roll onto a guest house flee-ridden bed and laugh. How our bicycles were like our children, how we were like the children of the Vietnamese people who ran out of their houses to help us. How they were like our children, curious about lip balm and bicycle tools, curious about Rupert's height and my blond hair. How my diabetes was like a third character. Like the questioner or Adversary—the "angel who instigates tests upon humankind" or at least, on these two humans.

The Ngang Pass, Vietnam, September 18

Sweat, a tunnel, shivering, my clothes glued to skin, my tongue sticky-sweet and Rupert in the distance, his hand holding me, keeping me from slipping, and slipping further and further down. His voice, firm: "Drink this, Yvonne, you have to drink." I blink and my eyes take in his large frame standing over me, his face shining, brow creased, above him the mosquito net, below me, damp bed sheets. *Whose bed? Where am I?* I sit up, lie back down, sit up and push Rupert aside: "We have to get going! Why did you let me sleep so long!?" A haze of dizziness, a rush of hot blood, followed by shivers, a cold sweat.

Minutes pass. Rupert, stung by my confused rage, packs. I sit slumped on the bed, waiting for the world to return to me. We are in a guest house by the side of the road. Today we will cycle to Dong Hoi. We have a mountain-pass to climb. Yesterday's dinner, gritty with pig fat, wasn't enough. It wasn't enough and I didn't wake myself in the night so my sugars sat low, adrenalin pumping all night.

I sit up again. Rupert hovers, almost ready to go. I loiter, incapable of more than sitting in wet sheets, shivering as the day reaches 30°s and humidity seeps in. I am hunger. Hunger that numbs my tongue, my lips, the tip of my nose. He comes back to me, holds my clothes out, and helps me up.

"Come on, let's get you some breakfast."

My ability to forget I had diabetes delighted my dad when I was a kid. We'd be driving to Edmonton from Sherwood Park for dinner and have to turn

around because I'd forgotten my insulin. My dad would be quietly pleased, say, "Well, I guess we'll be a bit late." He'd smile at my mom who would mutter something about responsibility. Years later, he said, "I was relieved you could forget. That you weren't somehow marked by it in every way."

Rupert's Side of the Story

Yvonne's sugars had bounced around when we travelled in Japan at the end of August. She kept having fast lows, and fought help. She'd zone out and then just wake up, so this morning's low didn't surprise me, nor did her response.

Our room near the Ngang Pass had the usual twin beds so by morning we were sleeping separately. At some point in the night, I'd moved. When I woke, I checked on her immediately. Her skin was covered in sweat.

"Yvonne," I said, "you need to drink this." She was so low, I worried she'd choke on the yogurt drink. She didn't want to swallow. She sat up and refused the drink. I didn't want to fight but I knew I had to get some into her, so I used my encouraging teacher voice. "Sweetie, you have to drink this now, your sugars are low." I put my hand on her back to hold her up and put the straw in her mouth. "Just take one sip. Good. Now another sip." She was incoherent and sweaty and kept trying to swat me away but it didn't take long for the sugar in the yogurt to hit her system. She was suddenly awake and hungry. Both worried and miffed. I gave her a piece of PowerBar. Then she was yelling at me: "Why did you let us sleep in?" I turned my back and started packing, then gave her another yogurt drink. She was behaving as she had earlier. Once she was really awake and conscious we had a breakfast of bread and peanut butter and packed up.

She was cold, so we sat in the sun outside. For a brief moment I panicked. I was also frustrated but remained calm so she'd drink. We never wanted to eat those PowerBars. They left us thirsty, but they seemed like a good idea in the winter in Japan.

My specialist says that hypoglycemia deprives the brain of its only nutrient, glucose, rendering the diabetic truly impaired. "Did you have glucagon?" he asks. Glucagon is an injectable cure for extreme lows. No, we didn't. I'd not heard of such a thing until I was pregnant, seven years later. We did have a tube of edible glucose though, but never used it.

Vinh to Ha Tinh, Vietnam, September 16

Riding out of Vinh we stop on a bridge and watch a small fishing boat float over what looks like a flooded rice field. The fisherman, standing, face sheltered by a straw hat, casts his net then pushes himself downstream with a pole. For me this is the quintessential image of Vietnam: boat and man mirrored in the water, silence around them.

We have gotten in the habit of stopping on bridges. Many have wide raised sides that let us get out of traffic and offer a good vantage point; we can see who is approaching and prepare. After fifteen kilometers, we pull over for a yogurt drink and to look for the turn that will take us off the main road. We plan to explore small villages and country roads.

"Hello, where you from?" a young woman asks, approaching from behind, her mother in tow.

"Canada."

"Where are you going?"

"We are going toward Hue. Today maybe Ha Tinh," I say.

"Why do you want to go to Ha Tinh?"

"We have to. It's the next town."

She must be about seventeen. She and her mother chat in Vietnamese, then invite us over for drinks. We follow them back up the road to their house. It is colonial in appearance with a small drink stand at the front. The drink stand, we have come to understand, is a typical addition to the front of a house. To make extra money, many families sell snacks, packaged cookies, Coke, water and yogurt drinks in a front room or garage open to the street.

"My name is Viet Ha," the young woman says as we walk.

"I'm Yvonne, this is Rupert." I pronounce our names slowly and clearly and repeat hers back to her, hoping I have heard it correctly. My name sounds breathy when she says it back, Rupert's soft and full of vowels. *Luupaaa.*

Viet Ha's brother says "Hello" as we enter the enclosed back garden with its wooden chairs. Moments later, her father joins us. He can speak French, German and Russian. His daughter manages English and her brother knows a little too. The mother is quiet.

"Would you want a drink?" asks Viet Ha.

"Uh, no I'm okay," I say, wary of taking advantage and of being taken advantage of. Wary of making an assumption of wealth. My fear is no doubt absurdly exaggerated but I wonder if accepting a drink means we'll pay for Viet Ha's college tuition.

She directs us to the dining table at one side of the room. Her parents and brother sit at the other side in chairs and on the sofa. She brings out a plate of grapes and sits with her back to her family. We nibble while she charms us with conversation, not wanting to share us, just yet, with her waiting family. She has done some modeling, she says, handing Rupert some plasticized photos. She also loves to sing.

Once she's told us her life story, she relaxes and moves aside so we can chat with everyone. Her father worked as an engineer. In his youth, the Soviet and Vietnamese government had exchanges and he was able to study in Moscow. He still travels for business.

"In fact," he says, leaning forward, "I am one of few to travel."

This is the first Vietnamese family we've met who can afford to fly in and out of the country regularly. I believe he and his family represent the Vietnamese middle class. Even so, they still have the small shop at the front of their house.

Viet Ha offers Rupert a Coke. There is no mention of money, only kindness and curiosity about our plans. After an hour we are anxious to get back on the road and tell the family that we must be on our way; we have far to go.

Before we leave I give Canada tattoos to Viet Ha and her brother, and Canada pins to her parents. Most children in Vietnam covet pens and pencils which would have broken in our bags. The pins and tattoos are all we have, though I feel a little embarrassed by them. Easy to carry, they always seem inadequate. We exchange addresses. While I write ours on a piece of paper, the family talks excitedly. A few minutes later the brother runs inside and returns with a folded Vietnamese flag and offers it to us. The yellow star on a bright red background will represent this family to us. Suddenly, we have friends nearby.

I did not want to cycle through villages and cities collecting experiences like a beachcomber gathering shells and scraps of metal. I wanted to meet people. I wanted to be ignored. Accuse me of being too simple? I accuse myself. Now, bombings in Bangkok. Terrorism in Paris. Violence in the U.S. Still wealth flares around poverty. Bike lanes in Asia. The world changes while I hunch over memories and doubt. I know I was both subject and object. I observed; I was observed. I judged; I was judged.

Were we manifestations of globalization: two white twenty-somethings on bicycles in Vietnam, Laos, Thailand, Malaysia, buying Coke and Starbucks? Our feet were rootless, we grew out of foreign soil.

I stop beside Rupert on the road back to town, "What's wrong?"

"My wheel's seized." He jigs the spokes and wiggles the wheel but it won't move. Then a few ball bearings roll out of the hub.

We have been staying in Vientiane for a few days and took a morning ride about twenty kilometers south to visit a park of enormous and varied cement statues of the Buddha. Now, some distance from town, we are on our way back to our hotel.

"Hmmm," I sigh.

"I'll have to catch a tuk-tuk."

I tilt my head and look around and feel sure that I know the way. I tell Rupert I can get back on my own. We walk for a bit, until we come to a strip-mall of shops selling fans and other electronics. When a tuk-tuk pulls up, I help Rupert with his bike and wave him off. "I'll see you back at the guest house."

I watch the tuk-tuk shrink in the distance, then swing my leg over my bike and follow. I wouldn't have done this in Vietnam. Wouldn't have left Rupert a week ago when I was stuck in the back of a truck wanting to ride. But my bike is working well and on my own I fly. The familiar road whizzes past and I take in new sights: water buffalo, school children, the men who sell drinks from their bikes, ringing bells as they come near, people selling coffee in plastic bags from the front of their houses, children running bare foot and wild. I feel equally wild and child-like.

When I arrive at the guest house Rupert is sitting at the side of the road, his bike in pieces. "How's it going?"

"The axel's stripped," he says, shaking his head. "I don't know…" His voice trails off.

"Do you want to go back to that bike guy?"

"No."

Rupert works on his bike for over an hour, but finally gives up and takes it up the hill to the bike shop. I continue to sit with the metal bits and pieces, my shins covered in mud from the ride home. Suddenly, women appear out of the buildings around me dressed in bright silk shirts and dark pants, or long bright shawls. I hear a bell, *ding, ding, ding,* and watch the women follow the sound, their heads turning, eyes following a man on a bicycle. A large tin box is strapped to the back. He stops in the middle of the road and instantly the women surround him, holding out money to buy huge, freshly baked baguettes. I watch in awe, then stand, brush myself off and, keeping one eye on Rupert's bike bits, follow the scent of bread, counting out pocket change as I go.

This time I'm invisible, everyone tuned to the bread man. Usually someone forgets to move because he is watching me. Traffic stops. But not this time. Bread as a form of religion so the blonde foreigner is invisible. My friend Maria lived in Ghana for three years. She told me if on the way to church a group of Ghanaians saw her, they would go home. "We have already seen God," they would say. "There is no need to go to church."

On a wicker sofa, behind a row of salon chairs, I watch a woman cut Rupert's hair. He catches my eye and rolls his. After half an hour, the stylist has only cut a millimetre off one small patch at the top. Granted, she seems new to the job. I could have done it faster but felt shy about taking the razor off her. She shaves one feathery hair at a time, no scissors. The only blond hair she's ever seen, I think, or cut. Normally, Rupert's hair is light brown, but now is sun-bleached. He catches my eye in the mirror again and raises his eyebrows. I am also familiar with the slow haircut. In Japan a crowd would gather around my chair, all the other customers momentarily ignored, while the stylists threw up handfuls of my hair and caught it as it drifted down. The texture of my child-like soft blond hair unlike anything most Japanese stylists had encountered.

A sales man comes in. He has a plethora of boxes of hair and skin care treatments to sell. A tall, immaculate woman in her late forties clips in on high heels behind him and sits on the couch next to me. She has a cell phone in her right hand, long red nails and a calendar in her left.

"Hello, what are you doing here?" she asks, smiling at me.

"I'm waiting while my husband," I point, "gets his hair cut."

"Yes, but what are you *doing* here?"

"Oh, we're travelling. We've been cycling in Thailand, Laos and Vietnam for the last few weeks."

"Cycling?" She looks me up and down.

"Yes. We lived in Japan and now we're cycling. We'll go home in a few weeks."

"Home?'

"Canada."

"In Japan what did you do?"

"Taught English." The conversation continues. The woman has a polished intensity. Rupert rubs his eyes, enduring the slowest haircut known to man.

"My friend owns a school here. You should stay and work."

"Oh. I…" Oooh, what a great idea, I think quietly. "Where?"

"Just down the street. Let me call her."

She dials and chats, interrupts her conversation on the phone to ask me questions, or give details. "My friend runs an English school, one of the teachers just left, there is an opening. You would have to sign a three-month contract. You must call her. Here is her number."

I take the number and nod feeling deer-in-headlights.

"There is a pay phone over there," she points, "You call her, ok."

I nod again. "I'll have to talk with my husband."

"Yes, but not much time to think about it. You start tomorrow, yes."

I nod vaguely, find cash to pay for the haircut and walk out behind Rupert.

He looks famished. His hair long at the top of his head making him look like a little monk boy. Outside it is dark, so we won't get to see much of the town. Oh well, I tell myself, life isn't just about what you see, but also who you meet. We will discuss the tempting offer to stay and teach, though I know we won't. Every day we work our way down this long road toward Kuala Lumpur and home.

We walk up a long curved street to view the architecture in the fading light. I can see families with kids paying for a carousel and there seems to be a lot of touristy attractions. We walk around the curve and back up the street toward the pay phone where I call the school mistress.

"Hello, this is Yvonne."

"Ah yes, you going to work for me?"

The voice at the other end is determined that we stay while I am determined that we go home but come back in three months. She will have none of it. After hanging up, I relate the conversation to Rupert.

"Tempting," he says, leading me to a German restaurant we've heard of: something as exotic as potatoes for me and meat for him.

On Google, images of the town of Songkhla reveal beaches, an aquarium, a mermaid statue. But we saw none of those things. We stepped out of the threshold for a moment to explore another threshold. Work. Staying. The day-to-day of a haircut. We needed something more. We'd been away from home for two years, two months. We needed an infusion of that feeling you have about a place when you bump into people you went to University with, or know the best place for coffee. We needed to be infused with the familiar for a while.

I think we had become a resource, our language a commodity that could be mined and gathered. We were being colonized by the need for English language education. Was I tempted? Yes. All you need is a sense of welcome, a feeling that you belong to something larger than two foreigners on bikes on the reptile road.

Cua Lo, Vietnam, September 14

My ass hurts, my back hurts, my left shoulder is so tight my hand is numb, and speaking of numb, I'm no longer sure I have baby toes on either of my feet. I pedal and shake out my feet, or I try to wiggle my toes inside my shoes, but nothing seems to make a difference. My toes have fallen off. I've left them somewhere on the road behind.

My internal mutterings are interrupted by the sight of Rupert pulling off ahead. Thank god, a break. If it weren't terribly impolite and attract too much attention, I'd peel off my shorts and lie on my belly to give my ass the proper rest it deserves.

Of course, once he's watching me, I try to look energetic. I pull over, lean my bike in the shade next to his and step into the shaded shelter, adding a bounce as I go.

The roads in Vietnam and other parts of Southeast Asia are dotted with little gazebo-like bus shelters. Sometimes people do seem to be waiting for buses, sometimes they just look like they are shooting the breeze out of the sun. This shelter thankfully is empty. I'm in no mood to socialize, but also don't want to be left to my own thoughts.

"I'm pooped." I take a long look at Rupert and decide he is too. "How many days have we been going now? Perhaps it's time for a day off."

We pull the map out of a pannier, open it and try to figure out where we are. We reckon Cang is the next town, another twenty or so kilometers, and Vinh another two days ride from there. Another two days! We'd be happier resting for a day in a city centre where we could stock up on yogurt drinks and do some sightseeing, but neither of us wants to ride another two days.

"Maybe we could take a bus in Cang to get closer to Vinh," Rupert offers.

Technically, I'd rather not bus, but it would only be for a few hours and we would be less exhausted. I study the map closely and find a small, beach side town called Cua Lo. "Look, we could bus to Cua Lo and have a beach day. Just the thing to help our bodies recover—a salt water soak!"

Back in the saddle, the road offers bumps, green leafy trees, a few buildings of interest, a few cute kids running out of houses and driveways, a few picturesque water buffalo with funny gray birds on their backs. Mostly just a long road, lapping up the sky with its dusty, dry tongue. As we ride, I note the number of kilometers on cement town markers. I stretch my eyes along the road to see if a town approaches. At each turn in the snaking road I think it will be around the next corner, but no. I coast downhill, my legs straight, bum to the air, then ride up the next, coasting and riding and coasting and then, in a blink, we arrive in Cang.

"Don't the towns just spring up out of nowhere," Rupert yells ahead to me.

We stop in what looks like the town centre and market. A group of about twenty people mill about, their wares laid out on a few tarps around a clock tower. We've been riding a secondary road, so the traffic has been thinner. We lean our bikes in to each other and I dig for the phrase book.

"Bus?" Rupert asks an elderly woman in a bright red bandana, baggy trousers and shirt, her vegetable basket laden with bananas, her smile broad and welcoming.

She nods in reply and holds out the bananas. Rupert buys a small bunch and tries again. "Bus?"

A young man approaches. "The bus stops right here, where you go?"

"Cua Lo."

"Maybe the bus comes in ten minutes," he says, before confirming with someone. "Yes, maybe ten or fifteen minutes. For locals it is 1000 dong." He shrugs his shoulders, wanting to chat but unable to find the words. Then, from across the crowd, another young man calls to him. He nods at Rupert, eyes me and runs off.

We wander to the back of the area, away from the street, and find a food stall selling iced water and Coke. Ten or fifteen minutes could really mean anything. After half an hour, we begin to wonder if we really are at a bus stop when the banana-selling older woman comes over.

"Bus," she says, laughing.

I touch her shoulder and bow my thanks. As soon as the ticket collector sees us he says, "Twenty dollars."

"No, we heard a thousand dong."

He screws up his face at this, and comes back with eighty thousand dong.

"No way," Rupert shakes his head. "Ten thousand."

The ticket guy smirks and starts collecting from other passengers. We wait.

"Fifty thousand."

Rupert grudgingly pays and we stand as the man gives a small, rude bow before gesturing for us to bring our bikes forward. We squeeze onto the rickety bus, three to a seat. Rupert's legs sprawl, too long to tuck behind the seat. His left butt cheek hangs off his seat. I perch in the middle beside a red-toothed grandmother, her hand-sewn satchel of betel nut in her lap, a happy gleam in her eye as she smiles to welcome me.

"That guy so ripped us off," Rupert says, watching the ticket man gloat to the bus driver. "I'm sure he's bragging about how much he got out of us. We paid ten times the rate."

The bus rumbles and jumps to a start. In front of me, another red-toothed grandmother turns to smile, her three chickens rummaging around my feet scratching for traces of food. I smile back, then look around and note a young man with a pig in his lap, an elderly man with two baskets of hens and three huge canvass bags of shoes. Above, in the overhead baggage, there are more animals, produce, and bags laden with whatever other essentials the locals are buying or selling. The heat is unbearable despite the open windows. Dust from the road construction blows into our faces. We bounce uncomfortably along for what seems an entire day, is probably just an hour, and then the ticket collector yells "Cua Lo!" and jabs his finger toward us.

I drag the panniers off while Rupert and the man jump onto the roof to unload the bikes. I get outside quickly to catch and bring them down gently. As the bus drives off, the ticket guy silently points down a gravel road showing us the way to go.

I am utterly relieved to get back on my bike. Sure, we've jumped ahead a hundred kilometres or so, but the cost has been high and I don't just mean the fifty thousand dong which is a little over five dollars. The bus's rattle and grind on the body, compared to the lighter bouncing along on my bike. The jam packed seats compared to the open road, warm breeze and fresh air. As we cross the highway to coast down toward Cua Lo, I decide that we will avoid busses from here on. A bus is a dusty tin can while my bike feels more like a kite or wild horse. I pedal down the beautiful bit of road with a warm sea breeze pulling me along and feel a growing sense of excitement at the little resort town that lies ahead.

My friend Maria mentions "white person's tax" when we chat on the phone. "You know," she says, "I was the lowest paid teacher in my school in Ghana because it wouldn't have been appropriate for me to be a House Master, but people believe whites have money."

"However, I could have left at any time," she said later. "Choice. People born there don't have that. I wish there were a way for Ghanaians to come to Canada and teach."

Choice as a result of colonialism? Choice to inhabit, work in another country, cycle through. The means is what we have. But could the world open, could it be a two-way opening? Or an opening without sides?

Tha Khaek by bus, Laos, September 30

The bus driver pulls over onto a potholed dirt road in a Laotian suburb. Instead of a 7-11 there are vendors holding their baskets of fried banana or sticky rice, individual cigarettes or condoms up to our open windows. Heading north, I am aware of the Mekong River flowing south to the China Sea behind us. The driver seems to have stopped for the single purpose of allowing us to buy things or so we can cook in the late morning sun.

"Rupert, let's just get off the bus," I say, grabbing my bags. He follows, quietly.

The Laotian men on the bus must think I am an hysterical western woman, jumping on and off the bus and yelling at the tall man with me. A vendor nears. She holds a shallow straw basket of chicken skewers, but must catch the distraught tone of my voice because she veers off at the last minute, stands under the bus's open window and makes a sale.

"We're missing the roads, the experience, the possibilities," I rant. "We didn't come here to drag our miserable bikes on and off buses for three months!" I no longer care if towns are a long way away or if we have to sleep by the side of the road. I want to ride. I can't stand all the waiting around and the loss of control—over how and when we go. My body's a mess, confused by my sugars spiking and dropping, spiking and dropping. The lack of a rhythm to our days is taking its toll.

Rupert, of course, knows all this. My determination to ride the whole way clashes with his practicality. "If we know there's little in the way of towns, food, accommodation for hundreds of kilometers, we might as well bus and get closer, then we can relax and enjoy the riding," he says. "We've already paid to get to Tha Khaek," he adds a moment later, hoping to convince me. "We'll ride from there."

We arrive in Tha Khaek and seek out the best guest house on offer. Disgusting. My mood does not improve. The toilet is a horror. I stand in a stall, put my feet on the little foot-shaped platform area and hang my bum over a toilet bowl that was once white but is now a cracked ceramic shape with a giant hole in the bottom. Once finished, I dump a bucket of water down the whole and rush out as quickly as I can, shuddering. It smells worse than a truck of stacked pigs. It smells worse than a truck of durian fruit (which reeks of rotten flesh).

The room is large, with two single beds but there is just something vile about it. We've been staying in similar rooms for weeks now, but this one offends me somehow. It smells bad. Bugs inhabit every nook. A trail of ants crawls from the corner across the dented floor.

"Let's go for a ride," Rupert says, hoping to cheer me up and get my sugars down.

We head down to the front entrance. We can't even keep our bikes in our room.

I just finished reading A Tale for the Time Being *by Ruth Ozeki. The book is set in two places: on an island off Vancouver Island and in Japan. It is set in different times, in quantum worlds. I am home from visiting my childhood home. I am drinking wine from a cup I bought in Hagi, Japan, thinking about space and time. Compression and expansion. In the book, Ruth and her husband, Oliver, have a big fight and he calls her crazy and she calls him a loser. When I accuse Rupert of being scared, of not really wanting to ride anyway and he calls me reckless, I feel time compress and expand.*

I remember Rupert not always rising to my bait, staying calm. Always one of us was calmer when things got tough. Now we surge and crash against each other. My restlessness and desire for a different conversation. My husband (like

Oliver) is better at discussing things in the world and how they work than addressing the questions that swim around the heart, questions about who we are in the world.

Irritated, I follow Rupert along another dirt road. The town leaves much to be desired and my dark mood only darkens. Desperate to ride, I want to see the country, to let the spin and thump of my bike match my heartbeat and make me forget the impatience of waiting and wanting. I want something more than dirt roads and dirty guest houses. Something other than slow buses and sluggish blood sugars.

Eventually, my mood begins to improve. We pass rice fields and grazing water buffalo. I begin to look out of my own head at what the countryside offers: cliffs and mountains encircle us in the distance. The colours and breeze, my spinning legs are a great distraction. Our *Lonely Planet* says caves are tucked into the rock along this side road that cuts up into the mountains. We decide to look for them and stretch our legs. Relax into the journey again. The riding also lowers my blood sugars, which improves my mood.

We ride for half an hour along a bright red dirt road. Because there is no traffic, we can play, race each other, or pedal slowly side by side, chatting about trees and birds. Were there birds in Vietnam? I can't remember any.

Of course we can't find the caves. One of our key failings: we are much better at stumbling onto things than searching them out deliberately. We once spent an entire day trying to find the hiking trail to the top of the mountain behind our apartment building in Japan, but never found it. Then, a few weeks later, we went with friends who found it in almost the exact area we had hiked.

In our search for caves, we head down a trail of wet mud to a large pond, following the voices of children. They are bathing their water buffalo. They scrub the beast's sides with thick mud, and then shower it with grey water. Their voices encourage us along to no avail. We continue, go back to the main road and take a different path around the pond and, full of hope, see the underside of a cliff edge. I listen for the bats said to live inside the cave but all is quiet. There is no opening. The scenery continues to pull us along: bright green rice fields hemmed in by the darker green of arbutus-like trees and red road ahead, multi-coloured cliffs, like jagged stairs rising to the sky behind. We stop and decide to turn back. On the way to our guesthouse, we stop at a washing station and scrub our bikes until Rupert's nearly shines white again, and the teal of mine outshines its new dents and rust stains.

I did not come to cycling easily. Camping as a child I rode round and round, wobbling and unsure on a bike that was too big. Falling off while my more athletic older sister teased me for my lack of balance. How many afternoons did my mom pluck gravel from my elbows, pour sizzling peroxide? She would tut-tut at me for my wince and whine and my clumsiness. At some point, though, the beauty of the machine seduced me.

The noblest invention. The simplest, most pure creation of freedom. Once I would have thought if we all rode bikes and became vegetarian we'd be living in a different world, better, unrecognizable from the one in which we live. I am less naïve or hopeful now.

Recent events: Brexit, the U.S. election of Trump and the deaths of entire animal species make me long for my less-informed idealism. But I can't go back.

Georgetown, Malaysia, November 13

Archway layered upon archway down the long corridor of attached shops in attached buildings. The sidewalks almost match, one higher on account of decorative tiles that have been added at the foot of the shop entrance, an easy trip for a tourists whose eyes are on the streets, on parked motorbikes, reading a pen-scrawled menu in a window. Down three archways from me a woman on her hands and knees scrubs the tiles outside her store. Early-morning cool, still quiet. She sloshes buckets over stone before the hoards arrive. An Indian-Malay with a rich English accent points us across the way to an early-opening Chinese café for breakfast, and follows us in. He sits with a Chinese-Malay friend and the two of them argue politics. The coming election. Their language is a hybrid of Chinese, Malay, Indian and English. A man nearby joins in. Though they are not speaking English, not fully, I can almost understand. My ears are tuned to the complicated play of language, the way it sounds and then does not sound familiar. Like a well-known song played by a new singer, one who changes the rhythm or cadence. Or a song played in a different place, out of context.

Two men in their seventies at Serious Coffee are discussing the movie The Imitation Game *about Alan Turing. They are discussing male sexuality, how one could have seen himself as homosexual. How the other felt that what determined it was...I couldn't hear well enough, and I returned to my own thoughts. In the background one man's pleasantly low and nasal voice. The long loose white*

hair of the other. Their deep comfortable intelligence. In Asia we could not eavesdrop. Then, when we got home, we sat at tables in restaurants in complete silence. We had been in a linguistic bubble, and now we could not ignore our familiar native language. We could no longer tune it out. We could not talk over it. We could not talk over others talking around us. We'd lost the ability to tune out and focus on our own conversation. We sat in silence, listening.

On the ferry heading back to the mainland, Chinese-Malay read newspapers in Chinese, with English headers. I am surprised by the incredible mix of cultures. Do we have the same fusion at home? My point of reference has shifted to Japan, its seeming homogeneity. The unwillingness to accept that any foreigner who has been in the country all his or her life could also be Japanese even if they speak the language, even if they call the country home. I feel confused in Malaysia. What is my norm? Isn't Canada a multicultural country? Why then does this country amaze? I decide my reference points are off and culture is more visible here. It seems that all three cultures, Malay, Chinese and Indian have a place and position in society and in their own lives. I'm not sure that Malaysia's politics are as clear and simple as this, but from my outsider view point it seems that way.

The ferry pulls in to dock and we push our bikes off and after a quick look around Butterworth, continue to ride south. Having left an island, the mainland seems new again, full of small quiet moments of surprise and delight. We pass teak houses and later stop at a truck-stop where air-con, flushable sit-down toilets, and concessions selling fried food recall driving trips at home. Playing at full volume, Cher's *Do you believe in Life after Love* follows me to the bathroom then trails me down the road and through the afternoon.

I dreamt home. Home in the bent fingers of my hands and home in the cal-
loused skin around my sit bones. Home in the cranks and the brake pads. There
we spoke slowly and clearly to be understood but once we arrived home we
listened with strained ears to understand. It was our sixty-seventh day and we
rode 114 kilometres to Puala Pangkor. Sometimes numbers were a home too,
the cost of this, the cost of that, what would be left once our money was gone.
The easy answer was two bikes, two tickets home.

Ngang Pass, Vietnam, September 18

We hit the Ngang Pass and quickly spin into a leg-screaming rhythm. In our lowest gears we grunt up the mountain. Rupert leads, I follow. Once in the rhythm, I take a moment to look around as switch-back enters switch-back. The road winds up to the sky. On my left, way down below, I can see the South China Sea and in the distance China's Hainan Island. To my right, the mountain peaks escalate from lush hillsides in this narrow coastal leg of Vietnam with the Laos border a mere one-hundred kilometers west at its narrowest.

We reach the mid-way point, where the road momentarily crests, then continues up. I hear the loud rev of an engine so pull further into the unpaved shoulder and pedal, all my energy focused on going forward, on pressing my handlebars down to the road so I don't tip back.

"Hello!" someone yells as he taps me on the shoulder.

"Waaa…" I nearly topple in surprise. Gravity and weight pull me while my arms and legs fight to regain control. The bus ticket collector smiles, jubilantly at me from the open door as the bus passes and honks. I smile and then shake my head, quietly cursing, my armpits tingling from the shock. Rupert and I round the last corner just behind the bus and stop to rest.

From this height I almost believe we can see all the way to the Great Wall of China, while behind us stand the many mountains and few valleys of this small s-shaped country. We rest only briefly before soaring down, tentative about brakes overheating, to Dong Hoi.

I recently read in The Atlantic's City Lab *magazine that in 2015 only 2% of the population in Vietnam owned a car, while 67% owned bicycles. In the western world, owning a bike is a symbol of wealth and leisure-time while in Southeast Asia bikes are used for transportation. In Ghana a young female engineer has started a social initiative to give jobs to Ghanaians, especially woman, and provide eco-friendly transportation. She has designed a bamboo bike.*

We were the only bicycles on country roads, but once we entered small towns and cities, bicycles were everywhere. Scooters and mopeds too. Big trucks and busses, sure. Single-use cars? I don't remember being passed by a car in our weeks in Vietnam. In cities there were cars, but on the road?

We ride and ride and ride. Stop at shelters for lunch or snacks, buy caramel popcorn and ice cream at gas stations, fuel up on water and check that the coldest of the bottles rest against my drugs. I test my blood sugars at every other stop. My sugars are holding up, my blood testing machine, not so much.

It has an automatic feeder to send out test strips. I slide a button to one side, then back and a disk inside, filled with strips, rotates and spits one out ready for a drop of blood. But it's sticking. Instead of ejecting the strip into the slot where the machine can read it and I can place a drop of blood, it just shoots the strip right out of the machine. I wonder about the rain and humidity, if the circuits were damaged when my bike fell in the water? But the machine was protected in a Ziploc bag. So why isn't it working?

"I can't test," I say after wasting three strips. "Let's try again at the next stop."

We continue on, our bikes casting weak ribbons of shade behind us until it is past six and almost dark. We stop under a shelter on the outskirts of Prachuap Khiri Khan, a small provincial capital known for its seafood.

I nod as I watch the rain start, "Our timing isn't bad."

"Yup," Rupert agrees. "We beat the rain."

We're on a main city street and though nearing dusk, the light glows softly in the late afternoon, layering images onto memories of what I've seen before. The street reminds me of familiar small corners on neighbourhood streets back home or in Japan. A corner store or gas stand, plastic bags in a ditch, a wide shoulder with tufts of grass growing between gravel and rubbish. After consulting our Thai atlas, we decide the centre must be ahead and to the right. We race down the long dampening street, curve to the right, and find a guest house, tucked in behind the market.

As we enter, a middle aged woman with long wavy hair tells us to bring our bikes in. As we walk in, I can see rooms above along an open corridor and ahead of us a large storage hall-games room-garage-like space. We lock our bikes and immediately see two gorgeous Cannondales.

"Wow, nice bikes," I say as I yet again struggle to remove my panniers. The bikes look new and in much better shape, and much better equipped for long travel, than our rusty steeds. Racks on the front and back more evenly distribute the weight of luggage. Clipless peddles indicate that the owners are carrying cycling cleats.

We learn from an Austrian woman, who is backpacking, that the bikes belong to a German couple. We've heard about them along the road. Most of the touring cyclists we've met are single guys. As we ready to carry our bags upstairs, I grow excited at the thought of meeting this couple, of sitting and chatting with them. Of meeting another woman cyclist.

I am tired of lugging bags up and down stairs, of taking cold showers, of showering at all. I am tired of getting dressed and undressed, of scrubbing socks that never dry overnight. I feel restless and just want to go out and find dinner, I want to sit and share experiences with the German couple, but they are not at the guesthouse and it is getting late. I can't seem to shake my high-blood sugars crankiness.

After my cold shower, I don my usual thinning rayon elephant pants and a new wine-coloured tank top that I bought the day before, then follow Rupert down the stairs. I feel a little more exposed than usual, as the shirt is short, so my belly is slightly exposed, and I've gone braless as it would show too much at the back. But on such a warm muggy evening, I decide I don't need a long-sleeved shirt. As we walk into the guest house's front room, one of the staff comes over, a man in his late thirties, and gestures that I should cover up. We are running late, and he seems unwilling to try any words. He has a kind face, and laughing eyes, but is adamant. He points outside, shakes his head, lifts his own shirt slightly to show his navel while pointing at mine. I quickly understand, or think I do: people will stare, it will give the wrong impression. I need to cover up.

I shrug at Rupert, laughing a little as I run up to grab my long-sleeve shirt to tie around my waist. For my efforts, I receive a nod and a crooked grin, as we head out for a very late dinner.

By the time we find the market most things have closed, especially the vegetarian restaurant we were told about. Vendors are packing up their wares under the now steady drizzle so we return to the guest house where the Austrian woman is sitting at the huge oak dining table that dominates the front entrance. We join her and nibble on bread from one of our bags.

"You want noodles?" the woman who checked us in asks.

We both nod. "Please." Rupert picks out two noodle packages and re-joins us at the big table, coke in hand.

Two of the Thai's, who live and work in the guest house, approach the table, one of whom is the man who gave me fashion advice earlier. He points at the table and we all nod for them to join. I slip on my long sleeved shirt. After a few minutes of trying to communicate in gestures, Rupert and I realize neither man can speak. The older of the two, has an animated, readable face and active eyes. He looks over at us and begins a conversation, in silence, using only his eyes and expressions.

He tells us about the King of Thailand, gesturing to the picture of the king on the wall above, the most respected man in Thailand. He tells us in hand-gestures how the former king was loved by the Thai people because he was strict. He used capital punishment for any crimes—drugs, murder and prostitution. In silence we chat for hours. We move from one subject to the next. He can barely sit still as he regales us, physically, with stories. He stands to relate his own history. Pointing to his ears and mouth he shakes his head. I nod and say, you were born unable to speak and he nods. He points to his friend and shakes his head. The younger man, we assume, lost his ability to speak through sickness or an accident.

Despite being born deaf and mute, he communicates with skill. Using only gestures, he shares his beliefs and his country's history. We let him do all the talking, unsure of how we could get our meaning across to him, but confident we are following where he leads. We feel adept at communicating in gestures with bits of Thai (or Laos or Vietnamese or Japanese) and English thrown in. Occasionally he uses a few aides such as pen and paper for sketches and a photographic book on Thailand as well as objects around the room. He is particularly interested in connecting with Rupert and often points to him to ask a question, simple things like Rupert's height and age. He gestures that he wishes he had Rupert's nose, and face. Wishes he looked more like a *farang*.

When we rise to follow the Austrian woman to our rooms, our new friend stands, to compare his leg length with Rupert's, making a gesture to imply he'd like to be as tall.

In the morning, we find a note from the German couple, but we leave before they wake. I am disappointed, not to meet another couple, another female cyclist, but we are eager as usual to get on our way on our fifty-first day of cycling.

The same rain that we'd stayed ahead of since Vietnam is now alongside us. Pelting us. Restless, we argue again, standing on the beach about our future. Or we argue about our lack of new things to say about it. We push and pull at each other. Perhaps we are getting bored of each other's company. Perhaps weary of riding in the rain. We have exactly one month left. We fly on November twenty-seventh. Home scratches at our soft edges. Edges raised as braille, silent as rain, as language signed. Tongues held quiet.

In A Philosophy of Boredom, *Lars Svendsen writes "If boredom strikes hard, one is inevitably brought to an existential borderline situation where one has to question the nature of one's entire existence."*

Mountains, Northern Thailand, October 16

We plan to ride to Nakon Thai, stay the night and in the morning take transport up the mountain to Phu Hin Rong Kla National Park. Student groups held Thai Communist Military training camps there until 1984, when it was made a national park. After ten kilometers of solitary road lined with grass and shrubs under a grey sky, we turn off Highway 12 and stop for water.

"We are going to Phu Hin Rong Kla," I say to the woman at the remote food stand, pointing. "Is there a hotel in Nakon Thai?" I make sleeping gestures.

She shakes her head, goes to ask another woman at the stand nearby. We slump and drink water, eat dried fruit under the cover of an abandoned stall.

"Nakon Thai?" the woman points in the opposite direction, looks at her friend.

I scratch my head and dig out the Thai atlas. Nakon Thai is in the direction we should be going, southwest. The park is in the opposite direction, in the Luang Prabang Mountain Range. Those two words, mountain and range, paired with our growing need to keep moving south, gives us pause. We are in the most mountainous range in Thailand, with the country's highest peaks. At least we will continue to be, if we head north, toward Luang Prabang.

"It would be good to learn about Thailand's past," I say to Rupert, thinking about the Thai students, the pages of information and maps fluttering on my lap. I read, "The Communist Party Thailand became especially active after the October 1976 student uprising in Bangkok in which hundreds of students were killed by the Thai military…" I stop reading and look up, "I didn't know Thailand had a history of student uprising."

"No, me neither."

"Now it's a park. There is a waterwheel designed by exiled engineering students," I say, knowing this will perk Rupert's attention. I continue to read, but in our hearts we know we will have to continue south-west, not north. We know that we have to keep choosing to cycle on rather than get sidetracked. After our snacks, we agree to ride back to Highway 12 heading for Phitsanulok, about sixty kilometres due west. It feels lonely out here, I think, as we push on.

When we stop we lean our bikes into each other so they can free stand. What more to say? The guidebook offers a tiny paragraph on Lom Sak and a few on Phitsanulok. Everything is skewed in this book, nothing quite matches up. Suggested attractions are a full day's ride away and that southern arm of Thailand pulls at us. We will ride west then drop like a plum-line to the Gulf of Thailand.

What do we know of uprisings? Of violence? Recently a friend was beaten by her ex. Recently Nice, Standing Rock. Recently Paris. Sarajevo. Zimbabwe. Nigeria. The tar sands.

Is riding my bike enough?

The mist thickens as we push down the highway. There are fewer towns. We pass small villages and a sprawling resort tucked off the road. For a while, the scenery—rolling hills, green farmland and smallhouses—reminds me of the Gulf Islands on the west coast of Canada. We stop again under a beautifully carved gazebo-style bus stop and pull out our plastic ponchos.

"If the wind picks up, these will be no fun," Rupert mutters as he dons his bright yellow cape.

"Better than nothing," I say, head poking out of my army green shower curtain. We veer back onto the quiet road.

The ponchos help but are sweat-bags and I can't see more than one-hundred meters ahead. In minutes I'm soaked, my glasses steamed and dripping. We make our way slowly, then spot a small, decrepit resort with derelict cabins. The owner shows us the one free cabin, and we check in. Inside, the cabin is cozy with a bed under a slanted ceiling and a sitting area with a coffee table and two chairs. The porch off the back slopes over the rushing rain-pounded river. The dark water, the paths around the resort, the little broken statues and glass sculptures—all of it strikes a chord of chaos and familiarity. Run-down hostels and guest cabins with barely enough revenue to cover the cost of keeping them clean, let alone doing upkeep.

The rain that has been chasing us since Vietnam has caught up. We learn just how torrential it is walking to a small road-side market to buy sticky rice and beer to go with our leftover veggies from Lom Sak. In our small living room we eat, drink, play cards and sing old TV theme songs backed by a chorus of pounding rain.

"Just sit right back and you'll hear a tale, a tale of a fateful trip that started from this tropic port aboard this tiny ship…" Rupert sings, getting every word right, while I fill in with my own words.

We are caged in ribbons of rain until it's too dark to see, then hold each other on the tipping tidal earth and sleep.

In Thailand, Rupert and I began to relax into the rhythm of the road. We were less worried about what was ahead because we were in a more developed country, a country both of us had been to already. When it rained, or locals befriended us for a day or an afternoon, we took it in stride, we began to enjoy it. My blood sugars had settled into a steady rhythm too—lots of snacks, lots of water, big meals and they were predictable as the weather—sun in the morning meant rain by mid-day. Was I more relaxed because we were cycling more or because we felt more at ease in Thailand? We had become part of the road. One adapts to loss, war, grief, joy, bicycle seat. We'd not been in a touristy town with other foreigners since leaving Vang Vieng on October 7, and I wasn't missing it. We encountered wonderful Thai people and perhaps it was that shift we found reassuring. No children throwing things, no men holding out their hands. The people were friendly and curious but we sensed no underlying threat or confusion.

Vinh, Vietnam, September 15

"Sometimes the road is better than the inn"
    —Don Quixote

Bang! Bang! Bang!

Rupert and I are lying under our too short mosquito net in one cot because the second one sags in the middle. I've been keeping cool with the paper fan from the water puppet theatre. We set the ceiling fan on low as it makes an awful clunking that I'm convinced means it will fly off the ceiling and kill us. We've been listening to the noises echoing through our wall for over an hour. Voices, then fists banging on our cardboard-thin wall, and then the phone rang. Rupert answered and said he didn't speak Vietnamese. Now someone is knocking at the door.

"This place isn't safe," I quietly say.

When we booked in I had misgivings. We fought for the first time on our trip. Rupert insisted we had to be careful of money but right away the place gave me the creeps. The fight continued when we went for dinner at the hotel—the very picture of wealth and beauty—two doors down. We asked the price: $30 U.S. By comparison, our place is the town outhouse. We ate a delicious meal. I had some kind of paella. Rupert had grilled fish. Everything immaculate, even us. I wanted to leave Rupert and join the French family sitting at the next table. After dinner, we walked back to this hole in the wall, arguing.

Rupert gets up and goes to the door. He places his foot on the inside so it will only open a little.

From the bed, I can see the man on the other side, wearing some kind of army uniform, his shirt buttons undone revealing a white undershirt.

Rupert talks to him while I wonder what he wants.

Turning to me, Rupert says, "It seems he and his friends want to come in and watch our television."

I shake my head and roll my eyes, "It doesn't work anyway."

Rupert finally gets rid of the man, and we move a chair against the door. Back in our hot little cot, we both stew. He loves bartering for a good deal but I should have put my foot down and said no to this place. After our most expensive night in Cua Lo this is our cheapest at six bucks.

"I wonder why the guy was in army fatigues," Rupert whispers after a long pause.

I'm reading Ryszard Kapuścińksi's book The Other. *Often he quotes the philosopher Emmanuel Levinas who believes it is an ethical duty to approach, be open and friendly to the other. Here we are the other. We are asking the inhabitants, who are other to us, to open their arms and hearts to us. In every small way.*

What do we misunderstand? Colonialism and fear. Whose? We are not looking to control or take over. We are hoping to be welcomed…is that how it all started, explorers and settlers arriving. What we don't really know is how we are perceived. Not even on my own street am I entirely sure how I'm perceived. We each have our own plot of land. Each our own way of seeing.

Fragments along the road, Thailand

Blue-lit sky and the sun rising out of low cloud and fog. Rupert palms the pineapple we bought the day before and we settle on the sagging patio, over the river, to hack into it with my tiny pocket knife. That feeling of independence. No matter what, we have what we need.

Air heavy with humidity, we ride south on the now flat highway. After the last days of mountains and mountain passes I'm in high gear, revved up. Eat. Ride. Eat. Ride.

"Rupert," I yell, speeding to get closer and pointing ahead to an Esso.

I am addicted to the caramel popcorn from these ultra-modern Esso Tiger shops located in the strangest places. Though I believe it's wrong to support multinationals, and that we should buy at road-side stalls, I crave the ease and sweetness of westernized food. With my sugars dropping I love to indulge in a shared Coke and caramel popcorn.

Side-by-side on the cement curb outside the Esso, our legs straight out in front of us, shoulders slumped, Rupert and I chew on our snacks like we are kids at a corner store back home.

The city sprawl reaches out to meet us. We are back on our bikes when a truck load of young men passes, heading out to a farm for work. Rupert spots a gold-covered wat or Buddhist temple off the side of the road in an open field and shouts back to me, "Let's check it out."

Recently, I watched for the first time, The World's Got Talent. *Totally blown away by the strangeness of it—of people all over the world performing, singing, training parrots to ski, making animal sounds. Is this our new colonialism? The two hosts in Japan are identical to the British hosts, other than being Japanese. Perfect mimics. Also, a suggestion of wealth when we jump to* Vietnam's Got Talent, Malaysia's Got Talent, *South Africa, India. The rising upper class of the twenty-first century. One conundrum of Africa is we think it is a continent with nothing but suffering, hunger and AIDS. But there is also wealth and education. There are huge cities, masses of working people. It is the same with India. Vietnam in the seventeen years since we were there has utterly changed. Hanoi has skyscrapers. We could not go back and find ourselves again—could not find that rough road bumping toward the temple.*

Dong Hoi near the DMZ, Vietnam, September 18

We roll into Doing Hoi, not sure what we will find. We have entered the Demilitarized Zone of the Vietnam War and this fact sits at the forefront of my thoughts. A sharp left on white gravel, followed by a sharp right and we stop. On one side of us a mansion, turrets and all and on the other, a river. Dumbfounded by the beauty of the hotel, I stay with the bikes while Rupert bounds up the steps to check on the rooms. I lean on my crossbar and take in the market, the water, hazy afternoon sunlight and a few other pale faces walking by and checking me and the bikes out as they pass. I smile, wave hello.

Rupert almost skips back down a few minutes later. "Eight bucks!" This deal is wrapped in a nice package for a change. Luxury. Too luxurious for our bikes, which we lock in an outside shed attached to the hotel. We stroll the market and I lose Rupert in the throng, then find him chatting with our first foreigner since leaving Hanoi.

"Yvonne, this is Ann," Rupert says as we walk toward a café.

Ann is a British ex-pat who has most recently been living in the U.S. but also lived for fourteen years in Australia and a few in Egypt. She inspires us with her stories and resilience. She travels solo; has met and left friends along the way.

"Where are you two off to?" she asks over beers once we are settled at a riverside café.

"Tomorrow we continue south to Dong Ha, then Hue," Rupert says. "Eventually we'll have to cross via Dong Ha to Laos."

Ann raises her eyebrows and we begin to discuss the dangers of UXOs or unexploded ordinances left over from the Vietnam War.

"It is a worry," I say. "But if we can get across in a day, we'll be fine."

"So long as there's some kind of accommodation," Rupert cuts in. "We don't want to camp down there."

Ann agrees. She has also been avoiding exposing herself to explosive remnants. The conversation moves to other things: nearby caves, sights to visit.

"I may see you again," Ann says. "I'm heading to Hue and then down to Danang and further to what's supposed to be a lovely town called Hoi Ahn." She picks up her backpack and heads off.

I sit back and contemplate. Unexploded ordinances are a serious concern—they are the reason we don't camp, though the benefit of a nightly shower also does a lot for morale. Nearly twenty-five years after the Vietnam War there are still fields and fields of UXOs that children still step on when taking a shortcut to a friend's. In Quang Bihn province, where Dong Hoi is located, MAG (Mines Advisory Group) estimates that forty-six tonnes of mines per square kilometer remain. Many people live within one hundred meters of buried bombs. I know this because I read about it before we came and keep reading about it as we near the DMZ.

"Maybe we'll look into buses in Dong Ha," I say to Rupert who is daydreaming and people-watching, enjoying the sun.

What were my parents' lives in Africa? What did they assume? What did we assume in Southeast Asia? A right to pass through, though we were never sure. Never sure we'd get our passports back without having to pay bribes. My dad was utterly poor, out of money, but the British, I guess, manned the borders, and gave his buddy and him a few breaks. Was that colonialism or imperialism?

Was it him being part of the empire, or was that kindness? Luck? My dad's knack for talking his way into and out of anything...trouble, into the next stream of being. Rupert and I refused to pay bribes. Couldn't spare the extra money, though it translated to mere dollars. We came home to Canada with nothing. No jobs. A couple thousand dollars which would have been a fortune to our Vietnamese friends. A storage closet filled with things. With clothes, books, a desk, our bed. Filled with nothing I could remember needing or using. With childhood. With university. With early writings and stuffed animals. With music. With silences.

"I've got a flat," I yell to Rupert who is riding bumpily ahead along a ragged patch of road.

He circles back while I get out my pump and patch kit. As we get to work repairing the puncture, a gentle drizzle begins and a crowd of men and children gathers around. We patch the tube, put it back in the tire, and pump with our ridiculously small pump. The tire instantly deflates again to a chorus of moans. I look up and everyone smiles and shakes their heads in sympathy and comradery. We start again and find a second leak.

I hold the umbrella while Rupert files the rubber so the glue will adhere. Once the patch is on, we take turns squeezing it between thumb and finger. We want to give it lots of time to dry so we don't have to do the whole thing again. One man in his late forties asks where we are going. Rupert points behind, says, "Dong Hoi," then ahead, "Dong Ha." Everyone gasps appropriately.

As I begin to pump, the kids jump in to help but the pump gives up completely. Someone runs home to get another but it doesn't fit onto my valve. I blow through my mouth, trying to cool my face but steaming up my glasses. Rupert dismantles the pump and sprays some WD40 into it, then puts it back together. We try again. It is so slippery and loose I laugh, but finally my tube begins to firm up. The children never tire of us.

By the time we are ready to put the wheel back on we have shifted about ten meters from our bikes. The force of bodies pressed in to watch, has moved us; a small river of curiosity.

I am reading Ru *by Kim Thúy a novel set in Montreal and in Vietnam after the war. As I rode I imagined the people around me as farmers and ever-poor but actually the Vietnamese further south had a very wealthy upper class. The French arrived in 1887 but there was less French-rule in the centre of Vietnam where the DMZ is located. Kim Thúy fled Vietnam as did her character in the novel. The character says, "Only those with long hair are afraid, for no one can pull the hair of those who have none." Perhaps when my tire blew we were in a situation where none of us, neither the villagers who helped nor us two cyclists out on the rainy road had anything over the other to envy. We were near-equals though we, no doubt, possessed comparative wealth while the locals possessed local knowledge. All watched or helped with innocence, I'd like to think.*

Quang Tri to Dong Ha, Vietnam, September 19

As we travel further south, the Vietnam War becomes more and more of a reality. Old men and young children abound, with few men in their middle years. Many of the young men, the fathers of the children we meet, who themselves would have been children during the war, must be working while we pedal the long road of their country. It's impossible to tell if the buildings we pass are inhabited or deserted. Many are scarred by more than age.

We near the town of Quang Tri, a beach-side city that was heavily bombed during the war. Our map marks this town with a war memorial. As we cycle down the dry, dusty road toward the centre of town we spot an abandoned church, pock marked with bullet holes.

None of the doors, windows or interior walls remain but the scarred outside walls are intact. We lean our bikes into each other and stand in the eerily quiet church entranceway. The walls are stained brown. The Viet Cong hiding in this church were trapped in a shower of bullets when US forces caught up with them during the 1968 TET Offensive. I take a couple of pictures, feeling strangely intrusive. Should I be doing this, collecting images in such a place? Two young men stand in the doorway. They wear military clothes, though camouflage khaki, we have seen, is sometimes a fashion choice. We don't speak but keep each other in view, unsure of what to make of the young men. I walk around the hollow building, then step outside and back in. The men don't say anything, but stand together, arms crossed, watching. I put the camera away and nod to them as I move toward Rupert. We return to our bikes, continue to the main highway and south.

My left hip aches as we ride, a pinched sciatic nerve perhaps. We slow our pace as we enter Dong Ha and I notice a couple of mopeds following us. Rupert and I ride side-by-side as the guys on mopeds pull up to chat. Rupert looks over at me, his body tensing. It quickly becomes clear that they want us to stay in their hotel but we have already decided we want to check out one that Ann recommended. The men remind me that we are in central Vietnam, near the Demilitarized Zone. The atmosphere has turned. People are less curious, more wary. As are we.

A woman, standing outside the hotel Ann recommended, shakes her head as we approach, "No rooms."

We can see no one except the two men on their mopeds just behind us, in the shade of a tree. We are definitely the only tourists in town—but we say okay and try a different place. While Rupert is inside checking the room and setting the price, I stand with our bikes.

The guys on the mopeds stop at the side of the road and wait, arms crossed over their chests. Not until we are inside, our bikes in our room with us, do they leave. I wonder if they represent the mafia of Dong Ha and if their presence caused the woman at the other hotel to turn us away? I also wonder if they are old enough to have lived through the war. I realize we are not the first westerners to come to this touristy spot. I feel unsettled and paranoid. Dong Ha is the gateway to the DMZ where tour groups and curious Americans come to learn, first hand, about the Vietnam War. Hundreds of U.S. vets and citizens have preceded us searching for lost friends, or children. To make peace. Not to mention the latest generation of backpackers eager to see where all the action happened.

I am looking forward to the security of other tourists, people to talk to, other "Americans" to distract the Vietnamese from us.

Sometimes rain and riding its shadow, fog, so that we saw what was not there, missed what was.

In Japan I had a student whose father was in the Yakuza, the Japanese mafia. The principal told me to give her a passing grade. Cycling through these beautiful landscapes I was always aware that in my full panniers, in a zip locked bag, tucked under my clothes, was money. My pale skin, its sun sensitivity. Everything we needed, we carried. When it got to be too much—heat, squat toilets, young and desperate men, crippled men and grabbing children—we could retreat in a guest room. We could hide in memories, our thoughts fogged and thick around us, our bodies bound to bikes.

Taiping, Malaysia, November 13

Rupert and I pause in unison, and pull onto the shoulder having just turned left off the highway. Behind us a group of people in white hood-like shawls gather at the side of the road, beside a large decorated archway over a gravel drive. Rupert slows, then rolls to a stop beside me. While I look back over my glasses, I drop my foot and pull my water bottle from its holder, eyes fixed to the group behind us.

"Oh," I say, as the group turns and I see the skirts, the long braids.

"We're you thinking KKK?" he asks.

"Yes, how weird," I say. "What a terrible vision in a place of teak houses and new growth forest."

The group of white-clothed people all look at us and are in fact a gaggle of Muslim girls waiting, perhaps, to enter or leave. Some shyly smile at us as we nibble our apples in the shade across the street. "How funny that we thought the same thing," I say.

"Just another sign of our connection, baby," Rupert answers, swinging his leg back over his bike as he coasts off.

I smile to the girls and wave before rolling on.

I note the confluence of cultures. Cultures on other cultures. American GIs on the Vietnamese. Tourism on Thailand. The British in Malaysia. The Japanese in us. Why so surprised by those Muslim school girls? Just unseen, unconsidered, not thought of. We knew Chinese, Indian, and British. We knew the dominant

culture was Muslim but we had forgotten or we'd been so pulled into the colonial aspects or…where were the Malay? The world is more complicated now. Or I'm more aware. Just now 9/11. Just now Tsunami in SE Asia. Just now Charlie Hebdo. What innocence we experienced, naivety actually, when we saw those girls and they saw us. Astounding and beautiful, all of us. And the teak houses, the rolling smooth road, the scents of the trees. What trees? What birds? What girls.

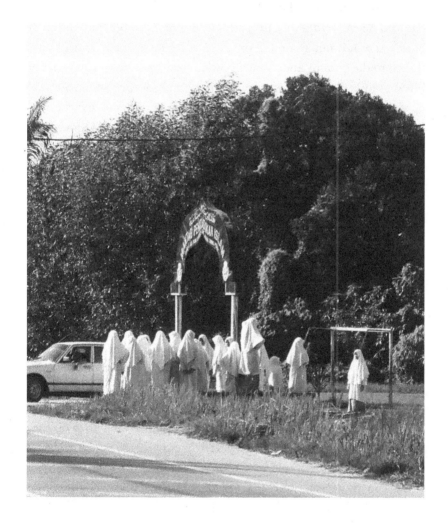

Riding North on Highway 13, Laos, October 1

We stop on a wide shoulder. Low trees and shrubs dot the dry rust ground. No bird song, no wind. Here, on the Laos side of the DMZ, the military dropped Agent Orange too. Trees are only beginning to rise from the once-poisoned soil. I root around in my pannier for food which, as usual, has shifted to the bottom under water bottles, road atlas, clothes and bags of blood testing equipment, syringes and insulin. While I try to move to the opposite pannier my handlebars flip, nearly knocking me and my bike over. I know the jar of peanut butter and three-day-old bread hide somewhere in one of these carefully packed bags.

"Aha." I look up at Rupert, who wordlessly eyes the road. "Do you want a stale peanut butter sandwich?"

"I really don't think that's a good idea," he says, in a more-serious-than-the-question-merits tone.

I follow his gaze. Two young men dressed like tribesmen, in loose shorts and flip flops, walk toward us, something slung over their bare shoulders. I scratch my itchy helmet-head and adjust the green bandana protecting it from the sun and begin to make my sandwich. A guy in a pick-up passes, turns around and comes back.

"Want a ride?" asks the driver.

I shake my head as I take a bite but Rupert ignores me and throws our bikes in the back, peanut butter in my pannier, panniers on top of bikes and shoves me into the back before sitting in the front passenger seat. As we drive off, I lick my fingers and turn to watch the men. Only then do I see their machine guns, but still...my eyes fall to our bikes lying on their sides and I feel ashamed, as if mine is glaring at me accusingly. I still need food, so fidget in my pockets until I find a plastic bag of body-warmed sticky rice.

After only thirty kilometers of cycling, I have been forced into a truck. I want to complain to Rupert, but hold my tongue. The machine guns may well be a threat, though they may also be twenty-five year old rusty remnants of the war carried just for show.

I read the book Little Bee *by Chris Cleave in a tent after nights of driving east across Canada. I willed myself to read it. My mother-in-law had recently died. The book is set in Nigeria. It is horrific. I'd sit in the tent into the wee hours, my son and husband asleep. My headlamp would shine on the blue walls of emptiness. I did not want to live in a world with such horrors.*

Who says, "Do not be daunted by the enormity of the world's grief." The Talmud I think.

I felt, reading that book about a Nigerian girl refugee whose sister is gang raped and murdered, that we should go and live in a war-torn country. That we should go and get our feet dirty. I was grieving my mother-in-law. I was grieving the bubble of the safe world.

And in that truck on a quiet Laos's road, I peered at my bike through the rear window and imagined it a fallen soldier. Bereft of movement. Fetched from the side of the road in a war that was small and in my head.

Rupert's Side of the Story

I looked back and saw two young guys approaching us with automatic weapons slung over their shoulders. Yvonne was preoccupied with getting some food into herself. She rarely senses threat when she first sees it. Her awareness of danger seems to seep into her brain slowly. Ten minutes, or half an hour after we've done or decided to do something, she realizes perhaps it wasn't such a good idea. Obviously, Nan, the driver of the truck, was nervous. He passed the guys with guns, then saw us and turned around. With his help, I was able to get the bikes and panniers in the back of the truck. Nan drove off before the guys got much closer. Months earlier, further north, Hmong or Lao tribesmen looking for attention, killed some tourists. I didn't think hanging around was worth risking our lives. As we drove away, I noticed my legs shaking. I wiped my forehead. My hands shook too. Yvonne's unhappiness was palpable. From the front seat I could hear her chewing punctuated by her loud sighs.

Is it true that I have no sense of danger? Am I naïve, always secure in the belief that I will be safe even if confronted? A strong will does not always save you, of course. This may even be the definition of naivety. Expectation over experience. Blinders. Necessary precautions. I am white. My husband, sensible. What have our parents taught us but survival? Rupert's dad travelled overland in a landrover to Bombay via Yugoslavia and the Khyber Pass and my dad by motorbike from England to Africa where he met my mom who spent her teens and early adult years there. They had some incredibly dangerous experiences, but survived. Perhaps their confidence, and mine, is bred from colonialism. My gregariousness begins to look ridiculous.

Paksan, Laos, October 1

We ride up and down rolling hills along the Mekong River passing houses on stilts, school children walking home and cows gone insane from the constant chime of their bells. We watch approaching clouds, ride fast to beat them but get caught in the rain. Rupert pulls on his yellow poncho and it balloons around him so that he looks like a yellow cloud on a bike. Excited children run to the street to splash in puddles and we come, we think, to Paksan, stop at the nearest guesthouse—white with blue trim—collect a key and collapse under the fan.

After dinner, we walk the town's dark streets listening to distant voices: conversation and evening TV, the clean wood smoky scent of a town that's no longer a village but far from a city. The resounding howling of a coyote from the sound track at the beginning of *The Good, The Bad and The Ugly* always enters my head as we ride or walk down emerging city streets. I look up to Rupert and say "ooo ooo ooo ooo ooooo."

People cease performing their everyday activities and turn to watch us. (I am Blondie and Rupert is Angel Eyes) then talk among themselves or wave and return to selling wares or sweeping dusty entranceways. With no streetlights, night swallows day, so no one can really see, from a distance, our pale foreign skin.

"The stars," Rupert says, looking up. "They're so bright."

I tip my head back, but my mind isn't on constellations. "Are you happy riding?" I ask.

"Are you still mad about going so far with Nan?"

"We could have gotten out much sooner and ridden more today. I don't think those guys were going to bother us."

"Did you even see them? You were so focused on your food!"

"You seem so eager to put your bike on a bus or in a truck. I want to ride!"

"Not true. I want to ride too. But there weren't any towns. We rode almost eighty kilometers today and I didn't see one. Those guys in Tha Khaek rode one hundred and thirty-five in a day, but we're not ready to do that yet."

"We could have stayed with some locals or found a temple. We don't have to always play it safe. Where's your sense of adventure?"

"Where's your sense of survival?" he counters looking up toward Ursa Minor and Cassiopeia.

Thomas King in The Inconvenient Indian *writes, "Throughout the history of Indian-White relations in North America, there have always been two impulses afoot. Extermination and assimilation." He writes, "The means of extermination didn't much matter . . . these were not so much cruelties as they were variations on the principles underlying the concept—survival of the fittest."*

Perhaps I've stopped making any sense. Diabetes and survival—is that what we are talking about? No, I am talking about indigenous people and the other, about war and young people, girls raped in Nigeria and boys coming out of fields with machine guns in Laos. I'm talking about "extermination and assimilation." Us on our bikes, the privilege of it.

We ride the outskirts of Hue trying to find Nam Giao, The Temple of Heaven. Our bikes bump lightly along the road, dirt-lined with thick grass and crumbling brick walls that surround the abandoned compounds. Hue sits on the north bank of the Perfume River and lies at the centre of Vietnam about nine-hundred kilometers north of Ho Chi Minh City and eight-hundred kilometers south of Hanoi. Eight hundred kilometres is a nice number, when you consider that we two-wheeled it.

We have been staying in Hue, so our bikes are unloaded, we are exploring.

"Hello, you from Canada?" yells a clean-shaven man with a slight moustache. "My uncle lives in Quebec. Where you from?"

The man pulls up alongside me on a tan moped and introduces himself as Yung. He then falls back to chat with Rupert.

Hue was once the cultural capital of Vietnam but in 1968, three years into the war, its citadel became the key location of the TET offensive, one of the worst battles of the war. Tet is the Lunar New Year in Vietnam and during the war it was the day the communists invaded most of the provincial capitals.

Yung rides with us to Nam Giao, but the gates are closed. He shrugs and tells us we can get into the tomb of Minh Mang for free, as his nephew works there. We agree and follow him.

When we arrive, it's also closed. There are no ticket collectors to take money. Pine forests surround the tomb grounds and in a courtyard life-sized statues of Mandarin soldiers, elephants and lions guard in a chess-board formation. Some of the statues represent military guards while others represent the people of court. The temple was completed in 1843 by a Chinese-appointed emperor, Minh Mang's replacement.

After Minh Mang's tomb, Yung leads us to his village for lunch and tea. Our bikes slip on the unpaved road that follows along the Perfume River. I spot houses tucked in among the trees and boats dotting the river. Fishing and farming appear to be the main industries. We pass several houses with the familiar front-door concessions on the way to Yung's large property nestled in the trees and surrounded by a breeze-block wall.

We pull up three chairs on the cement veranda while Yung's wife prepares lunch. Three of his four children come out to see us, as well as his wife and a young man who assists her. We drink lemon juice and Jasmine tea while discussing our plans to cycle to Lao Bao. Yung is excited for us. He loves our bikes and marvels at the freedom they offer: we can go anywhere on them, unlike Vietnamese bikes. He says he is determined to ask his uncle to send him a bike from Canada. In my opinion, the Chinese-made bikes the Vietnamese ride are much more suitable for their purposes, but I say nothing.

The local bikes can carry a heavy weight and last for generations, although Yung is no doubt thinking of speed.

I'm thinking about the new bike on the old road and the birds in my garden. Thinking about connection and separation. Of wanting to be the same but needing the privilege of difference. What am I thinking about? Today the rhododendrons in the park near my house are an abundance of colour and life. Spring. On the news images of Nepal, post-earthquake. I'm thinking about that. Thinking about destruction and survival though what am I surviving other than abundance and a chronic illness? The chance of an earthquake that we all anticipate on the west coast, but are ill prepared for. Changing ideas and the rise of violence and fear the world over. Money and value and wealth. Of this country and its abundance, its terrible history. The first people.

"They only study in the morning," Yung says of his children. "My eldest daughter studies English in the afternoon. It costs extra money."

Yung, an English and Math teacher, tells us the government supplements his income with bags of rice that his family eats, trades for other food items or sells at the village market. According to my *Lonely Planet* and Yung the average income in Vietnam is $215 USD a month and 55% of this income goes toward food. While the country is poor, education is important. In fact, the overall literacy rate in Vietnam in 1999 is 88% while the literacy rate of men is 92%. In Canada the overall rate is 96%.

After lunch, Yung shows us the world atlas a British couple sent to him. We flip through colour photos of different cities around the world. The thank you card tucked inside lets us know we aren't the first tourists he has befriended. I relax even more. I understand the prestige that comes with this atlas, and being a guide to friendly tourists. Often Japanese people would befriend foreigners for the gossip it created when they were seen with a tall fair *gaijin*. Not only did their English improve, but they became the envy of their friends, telling stories of what their *gaijin* ate, wore and how they lived. We are visible minorities but of the rare privileged variety.

While Yung and I chat, Rupert entertains the youngest son by snapping his fingers and clapping his hands so fast that, to the boy, it looks like magic. He then uses his hands to show him the steeple and inside the church and all the people, sending the boy into fits of laughter.

"It is not so much the traveller/writer's retroactive imposition of an artificial order that I mistrust—for how else can the random data of daily experience

be coherently and intelligibly reproduced?—but the way in which the representation tends to be mistaken for reality, and accordingly, the way mistaken readers (and writers) are unable to adjust to alternative realities," (Jeanne Takamura, Traveller/Writer: The Art of the Travelogue *quoted by Stephen Heighton in* Paper Lanterns *(Palimpsest Press, 2006).*

We leave our bikes in Yung's yard and walk to the dock to take a ferry across the river to the tomb of Tu Doc. The ferry is shaped like a dragon with sloping roof and open windows. It costs us 35 000 dong ($3.50 CAD) for the ferry, but nothing for Yung. To enter the tomb tickets cost 55 000 dong ($5.50 CAD). Rupert and I offer to buy Yung a ticket, but he doesn't need one. This isn't unusual. Vietnam is a communist country so all national sites are owned by the people.

Thousands of slave labourers built The Tomb of Tu Doc in 1867. Located on the Perfume River backed by pine forests, the emperor's second residence is also his tomb. Once, he would have escaped here to write poetry. Now, it is his burial site.

"Bucolic," Rupert says with a grin.

"Gorgeous," I counter, nudging him. "Idyllic."

UNESCO considers the tomb a World Heritage Site so has provided funding to repair the buildings. Heavy bamboo scaffolding blocks entrance ways. We walk on packed mud, gazing at the ornate brick and tile buildings which stand out with their bright orange-tiled roofs. Most of the buildings have grown grey and moldy with age. Paintings, that once decorated the walls, are all but gone.

Like at the tomb of Minh Mang, Tu Doc's tomb has three bridges that cross a pond and lead into the encircled tomb. No one can enter. When the last emperor died, the gates closed forever. Yung tells us that the emperor alone could cross the centre bridge. The other two were for the military and the court. When the emperor died, his servants carried him across into the walled enclosure and the gates locked behind them.

"This was so they couldn't steal any of the treasures buried with the emperor," says Yung. "The servants would have been locked in and left to die."

We wander around, sometimes with Yung as a guide, sometimes by ourselves with Yung in the distance. As we cross back toward the entrance, the clouds unleash a torrential downpour. Rupert and Yung stand together talking about rain, how it falls every day for about an hour and then stops. As I walk in and out of a covered door examining faded murals, they talk about the travel passes the Vietnamese must carry at all times. I can hear their voices clearly but can barely see them shrouded in the fog and drizzle.

"We aren't allowed to travel, so if you are walking and people don't know who you are they will ask for your travel pass," says Yung. "There is fear that people from the cities go out into the country to steal from farmers."

Standing side by side, looking out at the river, Rupert and Yung move on to politics. Vietnam is still trying to recover from years of war. Yung firmly believes that the people should not beg for money from tourists and should not have turned to begging for American cigarettes and chocolate from GIs in the past. "We have to be proud of ourselves and our history," he tells Rupert, adamantly.

Yung tires of waiting out the rain, so goes to the ticket vendor and buys three clear plastic ponchos. Rupert offers to pay but Yung keeps walking toward the vendor as if he hasn't heard him. If we'd bought them, I think to myself, they'd probably cost five times the price.

Born in Zimbabwe. I can never get colour or birth out of my mind. The have and have-not of the world. My white skin. What can you say to the children of the world? What say to the Vietnamese father who wants the best for his children

just like any other father? Just like my father. There is no utopian society but in our imaginations. Nothing is ever equal. Not for women. Not for men.

Back at Yung's house, we drink more tea. His oldest daughter, about fifteen, is home from school and joins us on the verandah to chat. Rupert and I sit across from each other. He and Yung fall back into their discussion of begging when Yung's daughter leans in close to me.

"Please can you give me some money," she says in a soft voice. At first, her request doesn't register. I shake my head to show that I don't understand.

Rupert catches my eye.

"What did she say," Yung asks, glancing from me to his daughter.

I look down, then lean over the table and whisper to Rupert, in Japanese, what she's said. Everything slows down. I have no idea how to react. I'd love to give the girl money but I wonder if we have been set up for this all day. Her mother steps onto the deck and stands behind me.

"Please," the girl says.

She sits so close, holding my hand as if we are old friends. I am confused. Yung has been gracious, shown us around, fed us, let us leave our bikes and drawn us into the intimacy of his home and family. He's also been firmly against begging, but is this begging?

"We can't." Rupert says, looking at Yung expectantly.

"What is she asking for?" Yung asks again, then speaks to his wife.

Rupert frowns at me, then smiles, a sign not to take it all too seriously.

"Yes, she needs a dictionary for English school," Yung says after speaking with his wife. "If we could buy one, the whole village could use it."

Rupert and I shrug in unison. I try to calculate how much cash we have in the wallet we use for spending money, without pulling it out and counting. "Here is 67 000 dong," I say, placing all our bills into the girl's hands.

"We should go," Rupert says. "It's getting late and we don't have lights."

Yung gets on his moped to show us the way. After we follow him for a few minutes, he stops to give simple directions. For a few moments we talk about his daughter's need of a dictionary and thank him for the wonderful day. I want to ask how his views on begging compare to his daughter's request, but feel petty. I don't want to believe he set us up. I want to leave on friendly terms but feel unsure and deflated. I am also ashamed of my feelings. Rupert looks at me, a sign he wants to get going. We shake hands with Yung who asks us to send him something once we return home. I put a photo of him in our address book, on the page with his address and ride up the gravel road back toward Hue.

After the Tet offensive Hue was squashed by the Americans. Hundreds of Viet Cong left the Citadel and disappeared into the city, blending in with the 100,000 refugees. They took up ordinary lives as if they had not just left a walled-in battle ground that bullet-marked a two-hundred year old citadel. After living and travelling in Asia, I wish I could blend in. Wish I didn't represent something that intrigued and shamed me. I don't want to represent the entire Western world.

As we ride back toward our guesthouse, I wonder how any culture can really understand another when the people in each have such subtle and varied ways of communicating. Maybe after spending a day together, Yung considered us friends so asking for money wasn't the same as begging from a stranger. The fact that we barely had any money added to my shame and frustration.

I can't get out of Vietnam or off Yung's porch. Over and over again I circle back. I was so angry, but at whom? At his daughter for asking, at him for possibly setting us up all day. At myself for not having more money to give and for not

wanting to give any. What is friendship? Cultural understanding… were we
friends, then, and don't friends help out? Maybe I don't understand nuance.
We had a great day with Yung and his family. We never sent anything from
home to thank him, which really, was what he wanted. That prestige. The
prestige of knowing the foreigners, as in Japan. We had the prestige of being
seen as special. He should have had the acknowledgement of his own special
role. But we did not honour it. Too confused. Stuck on the porch, stuck in
that rain shower at the tomb of Tu Doc? Like his servants, I walked in and
have never left.

Phitsanulok, Thailand, October 17

"There it is!" Rupert yells as he pulls over.

Finally we can see the YHA hostel sign with its big letters on the tall brick wall. I stop at the wall and peer through the gate before entering. On the far side of the gate are lush green gardens and teak buildings. The chaos of our last twenty minute ride evaporates.

"What a place," Rupert says as we stare dumbfounded, leaning on our bikes for support. There are a few other visitors wandering around in loose, Thai market pants and flip-flops that gives the hostel an Ashram air. A young professionally-dressed Thai woman approaches.

"How much for one night?"

"You YHA members?"

We shake our heads.

"100 bhat for dorm, 140 bhat for private room plus membership of fifty bhat."

The young woman leads us down a rock path that ends in a cement pad. Under a lattice roof is the outdoor kitchen. "You can use the fridge," she says, "Also the microwave and stove for own cooking."

We follow her up to the second-floor dorms, which perch along a narrow verandah passage. All window coverings are made from old teak shutters and some of the walls were built from recycled teak doors. After seeing the dorm, we go back down the stairs, like rung steps on a boat, and around back where the private rooms, with or without attached bathrooms, are situated. Our guide opens the first room and the moment I see it, I am enthralled not only with the room, but the bathroom.

I squeeze Rupert's arm, give him a firm yes. This is sanctuary, a little more than the previous night's price, but luxury. Up till now, we've stayed in so many guest houses it takes very little to impress us. But to thrill us is rare. At six to ten dollars a night, certain guest houses stand out, either because they are frightful or delightful. The YHA hostel is unique in every way: organic in design and beautiful in its blend of rich recycled teak. There is an airiness to the room. I smell flowers and wood oil, stone and earth.

We urge our bikes down the narrow path back to our room, lug the panniers off and lock the bikes under an awning. I stand in the bathroom wishing I had pictures of all the horrible places in which we've bathed and peed. Then again, maybe it is better not to have memories of those dank holes. For the last forty plus days we've taken cold showers. Toilets have consisted of holes in the ground with a water barrel to flush. We've washed our bodies using this same kind of holding tank and a plastic cup, bare feet standing on gritty ground, or in mud or on slippery planks of wood. Some of the showers in our rooms sprayed beyond the curtain soaking nearby clothes and bikes. Every time we check into a guest house, we ask to see the bathroom as if we might turn down the room because of it. Often there is no other choice.

Our bathroom in the Youth Hostel is an oasis. The slate stone floor and shuttered windows evoke an inside/outside feeling. Totally private and yet open to the air. A beautiful, white, Western-style toilet and a sink. A shower head with water pressure. A long window bench opens to the garden, a place to put a towel or clothes so that they don't fall to the wet floor. I don't know what Rupert is doing while I sit on the bench, dazed, looking out the window until I look up and see him taking my picture. It will be a long time before I forget this small, private room.

At a table beneath the hostel's covered patio we order fried rice, an expensive and not particularly delicious meal that leaves me wanting more. In our room I test my blood and take four units of fast-acting to cover the starchy meal and gather our backpack, camera, insulin and *Lonely Planet* before following Rupert out the gates to explore.

The youth hostel is on a corner on the cusp of a residential area so we walk past apartment buildings where children play and women sweep their front stoops or sit in the shade fanning themselves. It doesn't take long to find the local vegetarian restaurant. Our place. We eat a second lunch—twice as tasty at half the price.

The owner is Chinese-Thai and has been vegetarian since the age of twelve, like me. She insists we try her homemade soy milk yogurt with toasted sesame seeds. With the first mouthful, I enter food heaven.

"How do you make this?" I ask.

We chat for several hours, telling her about our adventures, our cycling trip from Vietnam, and that we taught English in Japan. She picks up on our weariness and suggests we stay and live with her to teach her English. In return she will teach us how to cook.

Rupert and I gape at each other. The thought of never leaving her shop is suddenly very appealing.

"That is very tempting," I finally say. Our host doesn't understand tempting, so I say, "Oh, we would like to but…"

She laughs and pats my shoulder, as though I'm a child. "You come learn cooking. You love it. I go back to work, you two talk."

Silence overcomes us both. I play with my food, finally cleaning the small bowl of yogurt with my finger tip. I look out the window, watch the sun gleam blindingly off the white walls and white cement. I have no idea what Rupert is thinking. I don't want to look at him. The thought of not completing the trip bothers me, while the thought of staying tugs.

"This food is so good," I finally say.

I can see that Rupert is tempted too, but torn by the lure of home, the rest of the ride and all the practical considerations. Road-weariness, pushing our bodies and bikes up and down hills through sun and rain, has made stopping in one place—especially a place that is beautiful, authentic or exotic—appealing.

We continue to sit and discuss in detail where we've been. The staff stand along the counter and listen to our conversation. It is after two in the afternoon and quiet.

"Let's stay," I say, holding Rupert's hands, my leg bouncing under the table. He is tempted, I can tell.

Half an hour later we leave with a package of the sesame seeds and soy meat balls and walk toward the city centre to catch a cyclo to Wat Phra Sri Rattana Mahathat. On the way, we pass a small procession—some kind of vegetarian festival. The celebrants hold up posters with the green leaf we recognize as the symbol of vegetarians. This is the last day of festivities, we learn, and I can't help but take the marchers as a sign for us to stay. Not one for signs, Rupert scoffs loudly.

"Three possibilities… have always stood before man whenever he has encountered an other: he could choose war, he could fence himself in behind a wall, or he could start up a dialogue," Kapuscinski, The Other.

We didn't stay. How different this story if we had. I don't recall discussing it again after leaving the restaurant. It was one of those let's buy a caravan and drive across the US or let's get pregnant now and have five kids, let's rob a bank if we run out of money, let's stay in a $200 a night hotel with a pool. One of those kinds of conversations. Brief. Fantastical.

Savannakhet, Laos, September 28

Behind our guest house, the red dirt road follows along the Mekong River with a school, houses and a temple perched near the river bank. We slow to a stop when a young monk comes out and invites us onto the grounds, then offers tea. As we settle on chairs under the canopy of trees, Rupert and the young monk, Novice Sinnakone, discuss the river's importance to Laos and Thailand. While avoiding any physical contact with me, he happily slaps Rupert's leg, pats him in gestures of humour and kin, his dancing eyes matched by Rupert's. Like brothers, I think.

As we chat, Sinnakone passes me a school portrait held on two corners between his thumbs and index fingers. I take the opposite corners and bow. Rupert has been telling him that we were teachers, so he hops up and runs inside the large teak house next to the temple.

"Living quarters?" Rupert guesses as the young monk reappears carrying his study books. He asks Rupert to help him with his English homework.

As they work, I walk the temple grounds, then sit on a bench near the river. I can hear Rupert's voice quietly explaining articles and other grammatical points. Looking across to Thailand through the darkening trees, I wonder if the path on the other side is the one Tamar, my British friend, and I rode earlier in the year. That ride inspired this one. I contemplate the conflagration of time—how I could be over there and here, how I know that road so well, while learning this one. Laos is a tiny country compared to Thailand and I eagerly anticipate exploring it. Every day there is something new to learn or something to learn again.

As we ride away, I sense the familiar which makes the long road ahead seem gentler. Rupert is content, having had time to connect with another person in a unique but familiar way. We both seem solidly placed on our path, as we continue along the water-front, then loop back to our guest-house to join Julie and Nicky, two British friends we met on the epic bus ride across Vietnam's DMZ and border. Together we head out for dinner.

Sometimes I sink into myself a little and watch Rupert, an actor on a stage. If I could enter his thoughts, how different this story? His willingness to wait things out. He loves the attention, the brotherhood, middle child of three boys. Loves solving, helping, doing. Is sure of his decisions while I think of all the possibilities, the what ifs and maybes. Under the dappled light of umbrellas and tree canopy everything glows a little orange. Orange the colour of laugh-ter and creativity, of sunlight and a monk's robes. The robes orange because orange cloth is most readily available; it suggests simplicity and detachment from materialism. Through the trees, my eyes find the orange robed novices. Find Rupert in his yellow-orange cycling shirt. Like a moth, he is attracted to their light; the novice monks to the play in him.

Snake Temple, Penang Island, Malaysia, November 12

Built in 1850, The Snake Temple is dedicated to Chor Soo Kong, a Tao-ist deity. Inside live pit vipers coil around alters, shrines, incense burners and chair legs. Though poisonous, the people believe, so the legend goes, the incense renders the snakes' poison useless. I have to admit they look pretty stoned, barely moving in the hot, fragrant courtyard, up the stairs and spilling into and out of the temple, which I do not enter. Instead I collapse on a shady step while Rupert meanders through the temple. Around me vendors sell everything from snake decorated t-shirts to mini replicas of the temple and plastic drums that create a steady stream of chaos and noise. Vendors yell out what I can only assume is "Look here, Look here!" or "Welcome, welcome!" Irritating music plays from the speakers.

Nothing has reminded me so much of Japan as this place.

Rupert comes out and tells me a Chinese man tried to convince him to touch a snake. I rise to walk around while he sits with the bikes.

The back of the temple opens to a walled garden where the carved fish on the ceramic tiled roof are reminiscent of the fish on Japanese temples called *shachihoko*, said to protect the buildings from fire. I can't help but feel disappointed with the gimmicky-ness of this place, though I also enjoy people watching as well as returning to Japan for a short while.

Some days my thoughts wander or I imagine things that aren't really there. Doubt does this, weariness too, loss of courage. Some days on the road I see

monkeys that are in fact coconuts in trees, I see home shimmering ahead but it is just the road and the shadows of trees falling across it. Some days, on bicycle or writing at a desk I understand the concept of time as an illusion. I am here on my bicycle in Malaysia hearing monkeys in trees. I am in Malaysia eating spicy Indian food and also in Canada eating Thai take-out at my dining room table with my seven-year-old son. My taste buds don't know the difference.

Re-entering Georgetown, Panang Island, Malaysia, November 12

Caught in rush-hour traffic on our way back to Georgetown from the Snake Temple, in the middle of a roundabout with Rupert behind, the sun setting ahead, I feel my rear tire blow out. I pull into the grassy centre of a roundabout, toss my bike upside down and remove the tire. We sit side by side, bikes behind us, feet on the road, bums on the curb.

"We should try the PUNKU SUPRAY," I say. "That stuff Masanobu gave us in Japan."

"It's now or never," Rupert says, not really wanting to pull out the tube, patch and pump.

The day is nearing dusk and the light has begun to slip away. Traffic has grown rush-hour manic. The pressurized can which contains a sealant will both re-inflate the tire and fill the puncture. All instructions are written in Japanese, so I decide the best thing to do is hold the can over the valve and push.

"Yikes!" Rupert jumps to his feet as white foam spews out of the can, filling the gutter and road behind us.

"Give it to me," he says, but when he tries the same thing happens. Thick foam, almost dry, floats out into traffic. He tries once more but the can is empty.

"So much for that," I say. "Maybe our valves are different."

Since my tube has nine patches on it already, I decide to use my spare. We only have seventeen days left on the trip, what am I saving it for?

Once the tube is in and inflated, we ride back into Georgetown along the now familiar streets of a few days ago. Nothing looks the same. Little India has awoken after Deepavali. Brightly dressed women in beautiful saris fill the streets lined with book and toy stores. Dress shops sell more of the colourful garments. The fresh sting of chilies and other spices scent the air. After days of craving good Indian food our taste buds will finally be satiated. Our lunch of mild dhal was okay but we know this town can do better.

In a small café, which had been closed before, a young woman drops two giant banana leaves in front of us the moment we sit. A waiter appears with a platter of four curries.

"Vegetarian," says Rupert, and the waiter disappears, then returns with a variety of vegetarian curries that he plops one after the other onto the leaf.

"Rice?"

"Please."

He returns and places mounds of rice beside the curry, then a boy arrives with a pile of papadums.

"To drink?"

"Lassi."

"Lemon juice."

"Thank you."

We scoop up rice and curry with bits of papadum using our fingers. I try to use my right hand, remembering Indians don't eat with their left. In the end, both hands are covered in curry and sauce is dribbling up past my wrist. After discretely licking my fingers, I sip my lemon juice. The young woman at the cash register catches my eye and smiles, fighting back giggles.

After dinner, we wander the packed streets. I pause outside a toy and game store, the doorway filled with plastic snakes and shovels, and listen for a moment. Beside me, Rupert is talking about the colonial architecture of this narrow winding street.

"Shh, can you hear that?" I say.

We stop in the middle of an intersection. I stand, head falling back, eyes to the sky. "I can hear water." I look around for a fountain or dripping drain, but there's nothing. "Rupert, I think it's about to pour."

The eerie wonder of hearing the rain even before a drop hits ground. I grab Rupert's hand and we start running as loud drops begin to splat, splat, splat as though some child is tossing down spoonfuls of water. By the time we get to our hotel door, we are soaked.

Rupert runs upstairs for our umbrellas and we head back out into it. At the next corner, we take cover under an awning and watch rats race from alleyways into open doors. The streets flood. Shaking my head I take Rupert's hand and pull him to the next doorway.

"Up the street there's that funky café," I yell over the rain. "Let's go there."

We've eaten a big dinner and don't want anything more, but we also don't want to hide away in our hotel room. We order drinks, gasping at the cost, and sit back, the rain thumping off roof tops.

"I should have grabbed the cards."

The waiter comes by and I ask if he has any games. He points to a shelf in the corner stacked with all kinds of games and we settle in to a game of cribbage.

An hour later, the rain stops and the streets drain. We pass a few flooded streets, but most are just damp, as if the rain were a dream; as if this island has never seen water.

By now we are playing cribbage every night. Here we are on a holiday. This time, we are going to have fun. Have I mentioned the rats running into shops to get out of flooding drains? Here is metaphor waiting: rats and us. Similarities and differences. We are exploring what we do not know. The things we do not know are also exploring us. In Georgetown, with its British colonial history and tourists everything feels calm and familiar. The colonization of place. As westerners we feel normal. We don't quite fit in but we feel as though we do. No one notices us. That is part of it. Part of belonging is disappearing.

Floating Market, Thailand, October 25

Tall, old-fashioned buildings line the main dirt road of Klong Damnoen Saduak. The bus depot swarms with Thai and falang visitors; we are the only ones with bikes. The same plethora of banana, BBQ'd chicken, bread and sticky rice hawkers greet us, hovering as we fit our things on our bikes, ensuring rain covers are firmly in place. It's been drizzling steadily; the day has not brightened.

We cycle south from the bus and out of town following a sign to the market. We turn right onto a muddy road where Rupert spots a covered bus stop so we pull in for breakfast. Our bikes fit easily under the tin roofed hut, and we eat to the clamour of rainfall. It is nearing eight a.m.

"I guess we should get going," I say, standing at the edge of the roof, watching the rain come down.

We are cold and damp, but hopeful it won't last. The rain comes quickly, we are constantly told, but passes just as fast. Looking at the thick grey mist, however, I am skeptical that it will ever clear.

Further on, I spot a covered café along one of the canals. A man sees us and shouts out an offer of coffee. I turn toward him and Rupert follows. "Hello," the man says. "Ah, you are wet. This rain, it is an accident. You come in here and have some coffee, no money."

We snuggle onto a narrow bench beside a group of three women and sip our coffee. The women who work for the coffee man are the canal boat captains. It is a quiet day for tours so they are taking a break out of the rain. In addition to the three women and coffee man, there is a younger man of about twenty, perhaps his son.

"You like animals?" the young guy asks, pointing his chin toward the back of the café. "That is a criminal elephant," he says.

I get up and walk toward it. Rupert follows.

Between what looks to be an abandoned shack with a tin roof and mildewed wooden walls and a stand of lush trees, stands an elephant chained to a hook in the ground. The greenery ahead of it out of reach. The elephant stretches its trunk to grab at clumps of nearby branches. The ground and forest are littered with garbage, tossed barely out of sight. Most of the garbage consists of food waste and plastic PET bottles. We've seen heaps of discarded plastic all along the roads.

"Must be a rogue elephant," Rupert says.

"Maybe it's killed someone," I say. "Why else would he call it criminal?" Back inside the tent, there's a new visitor, a snake named Mr. Chuan, looped around the arm and across the back of the young man. I sit on the bench, trying to keep my distance, while Rupert steps toward it and after an encouraging grin, lets the snake wrap itself around his shoulders.

"Mr. Chuan weighs, maybe, forty kilos and can eat a whole chicken!" the young guy says as its tail moves along Rupert's back. The giant snake is now wrapped around both Rupert and the guy's shoulders. Rupert holds its head for a photo while I retreat further down the bench. Everyone laughs. I note that the boat captains move closer to me as well.

"You want to hold it?" the young guy says.

"No thank you," I say, bowing. The snake is finally placed back in its box. I relax and look out to the canal. The rain has lessened.

Rupert grins at me. "Let's go by boat to the market. After all it's a floating market. What's the point in riding to it?"

I shake my head at his exuberance and mischief. One of the women is already in her boat, digging around for umbrellas. She motions for Rupert to sit in the middle, me at the front.

"Mr. Chuan will keep an eye on your bikes," hollers its owner as we float off. We've locked them together, but left all our stuff. Perhaps we are taking a chance, but we either go by boat or miss the true experience of the floating market. No point living in fear, I think, recalling too late my insulin kit still packed on the bike. I won't need it for hours, but shudder at the realization I've left it behind.

Diabetes is a small fracture, a space in the body that doesn't quite close. There is no blame or purpose. It just is. It is an inconvenience, let's say. It puts me in constant doubt. Will all the parts continue to work? Is this a low blood sugar or am I just tired? Is this a high sugar or am I just grouchy? The way I live is shaped by it. Colonized by the need for insulin. Dependence on it. Will it lead to blindness or amputation? Heart failure? Everyone has the same odds, mine are just highlighted. But it is not colonialism. Perhaps it has some of its attributes: control, the need for control, a form of violence in the low and high sugar. Perhaps I am the imperial colonizer. I decide when to influence blood sugars with insulin and with food. I am trying to rule the diabetes; the body merely the fought-over colony.

We paddle down the narrow highway of water, still a distance from the market and when the rain starts, we put up the umbrellas; our captain dons her pointed hat. Bright pink flowers, perhaps wild roses and wide-fingered palm leaves stretch toward the canal. The river is quiet but for the swish of the paddle and sound of wind in the trees. As we get closer, I see ahead small clusters of boats moored outside the canal-facing shop fronts and living rooms of the sellers. Batik rayon and silk dresses, shirts, boxers and pants are displayed. A woman approaches us in a boat filled with spices in ten-pack bags. We buy two and continue on. Now it looks like rush hour—brightly decorated umbrellas held high in a multitude of boats. All the captains are women, some of the boats floating shops. On the right a large building houses the main river-side market. Clusters of tourists stand on its covered patio pointing down at those of us on water. On the lower level of the building, people stand by river's-edge to make purchases or re-load their floating stalls.

I love the look of the large market but without my insulin I can't satisfy the many cravings it invokes, so we stay in the boat. I can smell all manner of delicious foods—their scents float from the market kitchens out over the water. I want to hop off the boat and wander inside, but we keep floating. As we glide past the outside deck, I catch the eye of a tall blond man, looking out appraisingly at the boats. He nods at me and I wonder if he is eating something wonderful and savoury and if he has a warm dry car to get into.

As we move away from the large market, I spot a shop selling hats like our captain's, painted with scenes of the country in bright colours. They look like gardeners' camouflage caps made from woven reeds. I decide I would like one for my mom.

"How are we going to carry it?" Rupert asks.

"I can put it in a plastic bag and strap it to the back of my bike. I'll ship it in the next town."

Rupert rolls his eyes while I try on several varieties. I want him to give a clear and enthusiastic opinion so keep looking at him for a nod or head shake. Finally he helps me choose one. "I hope she'll wear it," I say. "Though if she doesn't it could hang on a wall."

"How much?" I ask the vendor.

"500 bhat."

"Too much, 200."

The woman makes air-sucking tut-tut sounds with her lips and shakes her head.

"Okay, how much," I ask again. Our captain's normally serene face is now animated; her eyes sparkle and her lips part in a wide smile.

"300" the vendor counters.

"Okay," I say, "250."

The woman nods in agreement and I hand over the money and ask for a bag, pointing at the rain.

We pass vendors selling wood statues, cotton hats, baby clothes and felt dolls, things we've seen in every market since Danang. Viewing the scene and activity from the boat is the real novelty and attraction. After squeezing through a thick cluster of boats and umbrellas, we head back, circling to the end and then paddling up the other side. We hit a secluded spot where a huge tree dangles over the canal giving shelter from rain. Our captain paddles under the foliage to join a few of her friends, other boat captains, who are eating bananas out of the rain. After a short discussion, they pass some bananas to Rupert.

"How much?" I offer, but they all shake their heads and laugh.

At home my mom will put this hat in a cupboard for display. Of course she won't wear it. Too beautiful. I'm trying to be practical and whimsical at once. Whimsy seems to have won.

At home, too, I will have surgery to unlock my right thumb, the internal workings swollen and seized from over use. Hands hooked to handlebars, thumbs bent and holding. I will arrive home with a swollen middle finger, also on my right hand, from a fall on sea anemones. My doctors will tell me to stay put for a while. Get blood sugars under control, put on some weight. Stop moving.

We cycle to Tha Chang and stop at the side of the road to hitchhike. Our bones are weary: my hands won't hold on and my right thumb keeps locking in a bent position. For this, I blame hand-washing my socks. We need a rest. Behind us, in a pull-out off the road, a group of friendly women whoop and wave hello. We wave back but before we are drawn to them, a young couple stops and offers a ride. We chuck our bikes into the back of their pick up and bounce alongside them, the wind on our sun and dirt-streaked faces.

Phun Phin is a small rail town on the outskirts of Surat Thani, the last train stop for the larger centre. From Surat Thani ferries leave for Ko Samui and Ko Tao, so it is a vibrant centre where tourists pick up what they need before heading over to the islands. We hop out of the truck and back onto bikes for the last few kilometers to the city. The town's and province's name means "City of Good People" and we feel it, though the city itself lacks character; it's more a stop-off on the way to the beautiful islands.

We cycle down the wide main street with sidewalks and concrete buildings on either side. After getting directions to the hospital, we ride there first, hoping for a new blood testing machine, manual strips or at least to get my sugars tested. The city's main buildings seem to have been built in the 1960s or 70s: square concrete-slabs, with the occasional blue or green strip added for colour. The hospital's architecture is no different. There are no blood testers for sale at the hospital but the nurse tests my blood sugars and suggests we try a pharmacy in Hat Yai, further south.

We lock our bikes at our hotel and walk around to look for an internet café to email my parents about the tester. At one café we are directed to an international calling centre. After trying a multitude of prefixes to connect to a Canadian operator, and then trying our visa card, which doesn't work, we manage to reverse charges and call. From my end, I hear the operator say "Collect Call from Yvonne will you accept the charges" and my dad's voice saying "Yes."

"Dad?"

"Hello! Where are you?" his voices rises in excitement at hearing mine.

"We're in a city called Surat Thani in Southern Thailand. We think we're about five-hundred kilometres from the Malaysian border. Did you get my email?" I am quick and to the point because I have no idea how long the call will last before we are cut off. I also have no idea how much this will cost.

"I got it. Does the machine have a code or number on it?"

I read out all the numbers on the machine and he says he'll contact Bayer for me. The line is crackling but I can hear my mom in the background, so my dad passes her the phone.

How familiar voices embody home, the voices of my mother and father. It is November 1st and they are talking Christmas and New Year's plans while we are in shorts and t-shirts, the heat a white spotlight on us. After hanging up, Rupert and I walk into the city. We aren't hopeful about seeing anything too spectacular, but wander along the river and find a café to sit and relax.

After speaking to my parents, I am restless, a little adrift, unsettled by my blood tester and hopeful that my dad can get help so I can fix it. I find myself longing for winter, to be enfolded into the warmth of my family and home. At the same time, I feel determined to find a tester and keep going. After all, there is a new unexplored country ahead.

I tear up when I revisit this moment. That phone call home. What is wrong with me? Time has slipped through my fingers. And the body's aging delicateness. My parents are now seventy-seven and if adulthood exists, I am in it. I miss something from that time. Miss the wholeness of home. Then we were totally absorbed in what we were doing; from time to time, the world pushed at us. Some days we were pressed into all the complications of life at once. And then, I called home. Became a kid again.

Early morning, Surat Thani, Thailand, November 2

I wake with so profound a longing to be in my parent's kitchen, sitting at the breakfast bar drinking coffee and talking with my dad, CBC's morning show in the background that I am startled and wide-eyed in our dark room. I think of the immensity of Safeway, my parents stocked fridge and cupboards. The sheer whiteness of their house and the awe-inspiring breadth of their view over the Pacific, the ferries coming and going. Homesick. I am almost stupid with it so get up. I pack and we cycle, cycle and unpack; I cycle the long roads of this and the next country.

The body is an extension of the bicycle, the bicycle of the body. Years later, now, these two shadows—that shadow of my bicycle in the crevices of bone, in the sinew and cartilage of muscle the triangle shape of its frame, in the balls of hip socket the wheels, and in the ropes of muscle its spokes. But also and more so, in those same crevices and cells there is the imbalance of sugar and the need of manufactured insulin. The imbalance of how food and activity are processed in the body. There was another, secret, imbalance that went on. How to know the inner most secrets of the body? How to prepare?

Hat Yai, Thailand, November 4

Hat Yai is a sprawling, confusing city with narrow streets and tall buildings. It reminds me of downtown Vancouver. Old-style buildings are crammed in on all sides by newer ones, vendors, awnings in Thai and Chinese, movie theatres, a stadium and an enormous hospital. We cycle around looking at guest houses and then settle on one with my sister's name, The Louise Guest House. There are few tourists, but an interesting-looking night market draws us deeper and deeper into the city's core. We wind through the market and pop out on a quiet street for a late dinner.

The next day, a day to relax, we take an epic walk to the hospital, and from there to a pharmacy. The pharmacist, along with his whole family, searches shelves and digs around in boxes until he finds three boxes of manual test strips. I bow and thank him over and over, when in fact I want to throw my arms around him. Rupert shakes the pharmacist's hand and I pat his daughter on the back. We buy all three boxes. They won't be as accurate and will take more time as I'll have to prick my finger, dab the blood on the test strip then wait. After sixty seconds I'll wipe the blood off and wait another minute to read the result. There are two colour bands on the strip which match the ones on the side of the container. The numbers four to twenty-two indicate the level of my sugars: high, low or in between. I used these vintage eighties strips when blood testing first became available.

We leave the pharmacy and walk down the hot dusty city street looking for somewhere to eat. Once inside a café, I test and find I am a bit high. We are in rest mode, so I should have taken more insulin, though my sugars have been running high the last few days. I'm relieved to be able to track them again, but frustrated that they are high after all our walking. Why won't they settle down, I wonder, feeling the familiar tremor of guilt for not taking good enough care of myself.

Perhaps you are getting bored of this diabetes. Perhaps it is time to stop thinking so much. First, let's talk about sugar. My vision is muddy. It feels like I am looking at the world through a thick syrup that magnifies and blurs everything. My chest is wheezy, the high sugars affect my breathing and heart. I am clumsy. Awkward. I trip, walk into Rupert. I hook myself on some part of a door or on my bike. I fall.

My specialist asked recently if we drank enough water on rest days. Perhaps, he suggested, it is dehydration elevating sugar levels on rest days.

As we ride, we leave behind the last vestiges of Thailand. The road narrows and trees bow down toward us, as if to whisper a secret, as if to block the light. I feel as though we are tunneling from one country to the next. The road rises and falls like elongated moguls. Though low on energy, my legs keep pedaling; they pedal free of my mind, as if they belong only to themselves and the bike.

Sometimes you see a path and think yes, other times the path is blurry and the body unsure. Sometimes you are able to communicate perfectly with your body, and other times, when you should be at your strongest, the wires get crossed and you collapse, weak, lost, puzzled and let down by the very machines—the bike and the body—that you are trusting to get you through.

We are finishing lunch in a road-side café. "How far from the border?" I ask.

"I don't know." Rupert pulls out our atlas and examines it. We have no idea exactly where we are.

"Let's just keep going."

The matron of the restaurant comes over and touches my forehead then sends one of her children down the street. He returns a few moments later with a nasal inhaler that smells of Tea tree oil and mint. She demonstrates how to use it. It clears my head a little. She also gives me a small jar of Tiger Balm.

"You must rest," she says in her warm Indian accent. Dressed in a traditional sari in bright oranges and purples she symbolizes the country we ride toward.

I am a dreamer. Rupert, a pragmatist. I am idealistic, he realistic. Each connection with another human feels like an accomplishment with such potential it could save the world. Us humans with our ability to change the very atmosphere, ocean and soil. Couldn't it? Maybe back then; maybe not anymore.

Cameron Highlands, Malaysia, November 20

The town and its buildings shrink as we hike deeper and deeper into the forest. The sensation of cool air on the skin for the first time in nine months is something worth stopping mid-slope to note. Something worth commenting on as Rupert nearly walks into me, then grunts and passes. When we come to a rushing river that leads to a small waterfall and ends in a shady pool I am tempted to swim. But the water is cold so instead we dip our feet, sip the water and settle into the silence.

After a while, I say, "I feel a bit nauseous." Worried about my bouncing blood sugars I pull out my gear to test and sure enough, they are sitting at 17.8; they should be at 6.0 with all this hiking. My sugars are not responding as they should. Has my insulin gotten overheated? Am I fighting an infection? "Maybe I've picked up "friends"—Rupert's and my term for foreign bugs—somewhere along the way," I say.

I give myself a shot of three units and drink some water.

When my sugars are high and not responding to exercise or insulin, I really start to worry. The roiling sense of nausea could be the result of too much sugar in my blood, causing an upset stomach. Water helps flush the system. Walking helps too. However, if the numbers don't come down, exercise can actually make things worse. Each step I take on this short, uphill hike, makes me feel more dizzy and thirsty. The high elevation along with the high sugars make my heart and temples pound with each step. I am sweating and cold, sluggish and woozy, my over exerted body trying to rid itself of the excess sugar. If I have ketones, which is sugar spilling into my kidneys, the hike could be making things worse.

"I need to test my ketones when we get back," I say.

"Maybe we should head back now," Rupert says.

"Let's go to the next corner." I say.

As I follow behind him I begin to doubt myself; is it a mistake to keep going? Is the elevation causing me to sweat and feel light-headed? I am dizzy and shaky now, an unrelenting pressure throbs in my head and behind my eyes but I am determined not to miss anything. I keep hoping the fresh air and exercise will help me feel better.

We continue through the forest until the trail opens up to a field with a look-out station in the middle. We climb up to the look-out and cast our eyes over the green hillsides. I have never seen tea bushes before. They are a dark, rich green and even from this distance the strong aroma of tea wafts toward us on the humid air. I breathe in deeply. It is like inhaling a hot cup of tea. I let my head hang back and roll my shoulders then scan the hillside, eyes falling from tea bush to tea bush. "Is it real?" I ask, feeling like a wonder-struck kid. Is it real or is it a picture of something to make it look real, the bushes so green and perfect and strange.

Years later, when I am at grad school in England, a doctor (originally from India) says to me: "In the Western world people go to bed assuming their house will be there when they wake up, but in the Eastern world we go to bed hoping it will still be there. You are like that, Yvonne, you prepare but are never certain."

On November 16 I got an email from my dad with a code from Bayer to reset my machine. It worked.

Cameron Highlands, Malaysia, November 21

"Where's the toilet paper?" Rupert asks. I stretch my arm off the bed and pat my hand around the floor until I find the roll and pass it to him. He sounds strange. Cold, I curl back under the covers, but then force myself to get up, turn on the light and go down the hall where I get two more blankets form the closet. Other than curtains on the window, a carpet on the floor and our double bed there is nothing in the small square room. The toilets are down the hall.

"Have you thrown up?"

Rupert looks pale and ill. He nods and I curl around him in bed, his body cold and covered in goose bumps. We sleep but a few hours later he springs up again. I find our medical kit and give him some Gravol and we doze off again.

"What time is it?" I ask.

"Almost noon, I think." Rupert has just come back from the shower.

I bolt up and check my blood sugars, 18.0.

"I can't get my sugars down." I put my head in my hands and internally berate myself for sleeping so long and taking my insulin so late when my sugars are already all over the place.

"How do you feel?"

"Awful. Did you throw up again?"

We dress and walk to a small tea shop just off the main street. It sits on the slope of the mountain and sells tea from the plantations that dot the surrounding landscape. Neither of us has an appetite. Rupert is nauseous, and I am worried about my sugars.

"I don't have ketones. So that's good. Do you want some tea?"

He sips it, then decides to go back to the room and sleep. I take more insulin, eat some toast and tea, knowing I need to get onto a regular eating and insulin schedule. Then, I go off alone to explore the area south of town. We've heard about a famous guesthouse called Father's which has, in addition to a main house, nissen huts for guests. I can see, from across the street through a floor-to-ceiling front window, an arching stairway rising up to an open floor with marble-looking columns and expansive white-washed walls. It looks elegant and posh compared to our simple guesthouse. It seems expensive too, I think, as I look on from a distance at the outdoor seating area where guests are enjoying a cup of tea. Perhaps it was an English manor in the past. I don't go any closer, feeling under dressed and out of place.

I continue my walk to a school house with an ornately painted outside wall. Giraffes, lions, deer and the distant mists of Africa decorate the wall, hemmed in by real shrubs, hostas and ferns which give depth to the entire display. Could this be the British bringing the sights of another colony to this one? Around the corner I accidentally disturb a large white dog that sniffs my leg and leads me along a short-cut back to Father's guest house. I pat its head to say goodbye and wander back toward my own guest house and husband.

About a year after we returned home, I gave a presentation at a diabetes conference. A woman, about my age, approached me after: "I can't believe you kept going when your tester broke. I couldn't live without my blood tester. Why didn't you quit?"

"It never crossed my mind to quit."

"I could never manage not knowing my sugars, especially with all that cycling."

"*But we were doing the same thing every day, so…*"

"*Yes, but you could have gotten into trouble. And manual strips! I wouldn't do it. How could you adjust your insulin?*"

"*I had to make my best guess. I mean we were doing the same thing every day. Eating about the same. It was just rest days that threw me off.*" Besides, though I didn't say this, what would quitting have done? We were in Southeast Asia until November 27. I didn't know plane tickets could be changed. I didn't want to know. Quitting was not an option. Never imagined we'd not make it to KL.

Boh Tea Factory, Malaysia, November 22

In a long sleeved shirt and shorts I plod behind Rupert as we head down another trail, the scent of tea rising around us as we move closer and closer to the Boh Tea Plantation. The gloriously hot and humid day is still cooler up here than down at sea level; intermittent rain refreshes us as we hike. Rupert's stomach has settled down and my sugars have improved after a rigorous schedule of blood testing and insulin the day before. I woke this morning with low sugars and they have stayed stable all day. So, back to it.

The trails criss-cross down the side of the hill until they open into a mid-mountainside suburb. The houses of the plantation workers, I imagine. Despite the few conveniences such as grocery stores, cars are parked outside most houses and a bus goes by every hour or so on the main road, about five miles behind us. A sign points to the plantation and we follow along, now on a paved road. Shrubs of tea grow in clumpy rows all along the sloping hills to our left and right.

It has taken us three hours to get here and the tea shop will close in half an hour, so we hoof it up the driveway. After a very strong cup of Umph! so named because of the pick-me-up it delivers, we take the last guided tour of the day.

Behind the factory and tea shop sits an old English-style building that houses the farmers. Plantation workers bus in from nearby houses, and more are bused up to the highlands for work during picking season. Once picked, the tea is dried and packaged for sale.

After our tour and with newly purchased packets of tea in our pack, we head back down the drive toward the road. We've been hiking for hours and hope to catch a ride to the main road and the bus back up. We can't possibly hike the way we came before it gets dark. It seems risky not to plan every detail of every excursion but at the same time we know a bus will eventually come. Nothing follows a schedule, us included. We have water, PowerBars and insulin. We both feel great, though a bit soggy after our long tea-scented hike. Not being tied to our bikes now that our health has improved, is also a great feeling.

An Indian-Malay man stops and offers us a ride. Rupert and I squeeze in the back of his car, his small son sitting between us. He is tiny and fascinated by our strangeness. We groove to Indian disco tunes, trying to teach the boy how to snap his fingers. His thin finger tips bounce off each other without a sound while his father careens down the winding rural roads in his ancient Honda. At the main road we get out and wait for the rickety bus ride back up. A van stops and the driver reluctantly lets us in. My stomach churns as we wind back and forth, the driver in one hell of a hurry. By the time we wander back to our guesthouse for a shower, I am headachy and sleepy. I take it as a sign of hunger and am glad to finally, after all these days of lounging and carefully nibbling small amounts of food, have worked up an appetite and good blood sugar level.

We decide to try a vegetarian hot pot for dinner. Hot Pot is one of the famous Chinese dishes of Malaysia and our restaurant offers a vegetarian version. A waiter brings plate after plate of vegetables, mock-chicken and beef and noodles to our round table.

"What are we doing tomorrow?" I ask. "Heading back down?"

"Sounds good" Rupert says. "We can leave on an early bus, pick up our bikes and carry on to Kuala Lumpur."

"I hope so. It's been good to rest up here but I wonder if the elevation made us sick?" I've started feeling a little nauseous but blame the combination of rough bus ride and hunger. "Try this," I say. "It's delicious." Rupert leans across the table and from my chopsticks I feed him a piece of mock-chicken. "It's nice to fill up on protein," I say.

We eat until we are so stuffed we can hardly move. We walk up the street to the end of town, a five minute walk, and back again. I have major indigestion so we head back home and collapse in front of the TV with a deck of cards. There are a few other guests around—a guy from New York, an Australian who is meeting his buddies in KL and a woman from Vancouver named Jen who recognizes our Mountain Equipment Co-op tags. Who needs a Canadian flag? The MEC tags with the mountain peaks logo on our backpacks, fleece sweaters and even Rupert's hiking pants give us away. We all crowd into the TV room and watch a bootlegged copy of *The Matrix*. Everyone else in the room has seen the movie but this is our first time and Rupert is enthralled. The bootlegger filmed from the back of the theatre so we see movie watchers stand and walk in front of the camera, or hear them sneeze and crunch on popcorn throughout the movie. *The Matrix* came out in the spring, but wasn't released to Japan until September. By then we were on the road. Seeing it for the first time, after it already has a cult-following, I am aware of the broadness of the threshold we are in, that we are outside of our culture in varied and subtle ways. Many of our contemporaries have travelled in Asia, but over a few weeks or months, not years. Though I am fairly certain we'll reintegrate smoothly, I wonder if we'll be like young Japanese who leave Japan to travel and are never Japanese again.

Reading William Hazlitt's essay "On the Feeling of Immortality in Youth." I wonder what I lost in the mortal stamp of diabetes, always having imagined what it gave me, this balance of need and want:

> We are too much dazzled by the gorgeousness and novelty of the
> bright waking dream about us to discern the dim shadow lingering
> for us in the distance... we are like people intoxicated or in a fever,
> who are hurried away by the violence of their own sensations: it is
> only as present objects begin to pall upon the sense, as we have been

disappointed in our favorite pursuits, cut off from our closest ties, that we by degrees become weaned from the world, that passion loosens its hold upon futurity, and that we begin to contemplate as in a glass darkly the possibility of parting with it for good.

I also experienced something of that mortal stamp, a separation from our peers, as we sat watching the Matrix and our lives seemed to have diverged from our peers' norms.

Guest House, Cameron Highlands, November 22

"I'm off to bed," I announce to Rupert and Jen at about 9:30. Rupert will wake me for my injection, but I can't stay awake any longer. I change in the dark and shiver into bed, then get up and put my clothes back on.

Rupert comes in a few hours later.

"How was the movie?" I ask as I wake for my injection.

"Great."

We dose and then I wake again an hour later, and run for the toilets.

"Diarrhea," I report when I get back. Ten minutes later, I'm off again. "Vomited."

I sleep for an hour, run to the washroom, "Both." For the next few hours I run back and forth between bed and toilet. Vomit, diarrhea, vomit, diarrhea.

"Better test your sugars," Rupert says.

"They're 14.2," I say as I head out the door to sit on the toilet and hold a bucket on my lap as everything I've ever eaten pours out from both ends. If I can't keep anything down, I risk fast-dropping blood sugars with no way of getting them back up.

"They're coming down, 6.2," I say.

"Rupert, I can't stop. What time is it?" I sit on the bed, my head in my hands.

He sits up and pats around the floor for his watch. "Eight."

"I'm sure I've kept the whole guest house up with my vomiting." I lie back, dizzy and sweaty and ill. "Oh!" I head back out the door to the toilet. My empty stomach churns, my bowels pop.

Rupert gets dressed and jogs up to the hospital. Half an hour later a medical van arrives. A doctor tests my blood sugars, 4.8, and he and the driver shift me onto a gurney. As they lift me into the back of the van, Jen and the Aussie watch, concerned looks on their sleepy faces.

I am desperate. The hospital has become my only choice. If I could keep food down or gauge what is going on in my body, I might be able to manage on my own, but I am dehydrated and my sugars are dropping so low I am in danger of not recovering without an IV of glucose.

I jolt awake, as I am thrust onto a cot.

"Ma'am?" The doctor standing over me speaks English. I can't have slept long, but feel disoriented.

"Sick." I say and a paper tray is thrust under my chin as I puke yet again. "I'm diabetic." The doctor nods and Rupert arrives. I catch his eye and fade off.

"I'm diabetic." Now a nurse is putting an intravenous drip of Gravol and glucose into my arm. The thought of AIDS flashes through my mind— Did we bring our own needles? Where's Rupert?—but I fall asleep again.

Eyes barely open, I say for a third time: "I'm diabetic."

Rupert and the doctor are standing over me. They both nod.

"We are checking for viruses," the doctor says.

"We need to test your blood sugars," Rupert says, getting ready to prick my finger, his least favourite part of the blood testing process. He's using a blood tester provided by the hospital. My manual test-strips aren't accurate enough and my own tester works only sporadically at this high altitude.

"I can do it," I say. "Eleven point zero. That's good. They've come up."

"The doctor says you should take some insulin," Rupert says. "Some of your slow-acting to maintain your sugars while you get better."

I inject and doze off again.

Later in the day, I wake to find myself in a tiny single bed, the drip still in my arm. I haven't vomited for a few hours, but I also have not moved. Rupert is sitting in a chair next to my bed, reading.

"How do you feel?" he says.

"Gross. What a way to spend the night. God, everyone in the guest house must have heard me puking all night."

"Don't worry about it."

"How much is this going to cost us?"

"Don't worry about it. Do you want anything?"

"Water."

When the diarrhea and vomiting stop, the doctor changes the drip from glucose to saline and I eat a small sandwich and take an almost normal dose of both insulins. Rupert and I spend a second day in the hospital playing cards—I lie in bed, he deals and wins every hand.

"Can I get out today?"

"Probably."

"Do you think we can leave today," I say. "Get back to our bikes?"

"Tomorrow. You need to rest at the guest house tonight and see how you feel."

"But we only have a few days left." The weight of this statement hangs between us.

Your body goes off and makes decisions without your consent. The insulin you jab into yourself to stay alive works in ways you cannot always control. There is a balance. Imbalance.

Never tired, I was exhausted. Wired. My eyes began to ache. I was a bone rack. None of this surprised either of us. What surprised me was that there was a reason for it beyond the cycling, heat, and diabetes. My thyroid, which had begun to go bonkers pumping out thyroxin, was causing the restlessness, the nausea, and the twitchy blood sugars. But I did not know that then. We learned of my thyroid when we returned home. In the hospital in the Cameron Highlands we thought I'd picked up some really bad "friends". We thought we could get it settled, get me eating, and carry on. Though my specialist now wonders if it had less to do with the thyroid and more to do with dehydration caused by rising sugars and a drop in water consumption on rest days.

Not everything is in my control. I learn this not for the first time.

Longest Day: Thung Song, Thailand, November 2 (151km day 56)

Hooooo.

I breathe. My hands hook loosely on handlebars and my legs spin of their own volition. My eyes are on the road whirring beneath my wheels. The ditch to my right is full of water and the grass beyond is as green as green algae. The road: a cement grey snake with no head and no tail, just its endless body.

Hooooo.

I breathe and pedal. I sit and spin. I stand on pedals to let blood flow back to buttocks and to awaken my right pinky toe which has been asleep for days. Wiggling does nothing. Standing on my bike, coasting with legs straight and butt to the air, I am a speck in a movie; you can pan around me. See the hillside and trees, the tiny towns we can no longer bear to stop in, the road and the hills and rainclouds, or worse, the sun with its relentless glare.

Hooooo.

The best way to cope is not to count the miles, not note the speedometer or mileage markers on the road. Focus on turning the pedals and wheels, let the mind wander. The dogged mind comes back and sees we have gone one hundred kilometers. Sees there are forty-two more to the next town.

Hooooo.

Rupert is a speck of speed in the distance. Not too far ahead, but on his own course.

I distract myself by people watching, by observing people's reactions to us. Agog, shocked, amazed. We attract more and more stares. In a one horse town a man on a motorbike looks back at us rather than forward and nearly hits the car in front of him. When we stop at a store for snacks and water, people flock to see what we are buying, to check out our bikes, to touch my arm or hair and to measure themselves against Rupert's towering height. We should get a discount for pulling in so many customers, I fleetingly think, as another person at a crosswalk forgets to cross.

Hooooo.

I breathe as the sun starts to set and my ass and lower back thrum with each pedal stroke. I need to stop. I long for a Holiday Inn or Grand Hotel, a sign that reads "Swimming Pool" and "Room Service." Imagine pasta or sushi as the countryside opens for miles. Then a few houses pop up, then some shops and suddenly off to the left, a city. Nothing special, just the usual city on the outskirts of the world.

Hooooo

We cross six lanes of evening traffic to get into the city centre. Each large building looks hotel-ish to my weary eyes. My legs pump and pedal as if they are separate entities. I follow behind Rupert, wanting to arrive and be done but know we'll have to shower, dig clothes out of tightly packed panniers with tired hands, dress and go out to find food. Then we'll have to find our way back to the hotel, the room and bed. If all that isn't bad enough, diabetic me will have to wait two hours for my bedtime injection while Rupert slumbers.

Hooooo

Despite my weariness from our longest day, over 151 kilometres by the time we stop to look at a guest house, I am euphoric. Had I the energy, I'd throw my arms up and whoop, but I am guarding the bikes while Rupert runs in to check a room.

The room costs five dollars, our cheapest yet.

After cold showers we walk into the bustle of town to find food. I sit at our small table and say, "Whew, tired but I'm ok. I'm ok." Rupert agrees that he is too, but when it is time to stand up, walk, our legs are seized by ache and wobble. We throw our arms around each other, dodge market stalls selling everything except a pool, and arm-in-arm, tired but also kind of proud, walk back to the room and collapse on the bed to sleep. Rupert is snoring before my head hits the pillow. Bleary-eyed I wake, wash my padded shorts, take my injection, brush my teeth and conk out again. Tired, we sleep until eight the next morning and would sleep on, but for our bikes down the hall and the many miles ahead.

I'm thinking back to that moment on the bridge. Vietnam, September 12. We had just arrived in Phully and Rupert was in a philosophical mood. It was our first day riding out of Hanoi. Rupert said that life is about the small moments, and perhaps that moment—leaning on each other looking up at the sunset contemplating the road ahead—was one of those moments. How the miles have racked up: 3500 km. Numbers, as in distance travelled, are bliss to my husband. The moment one realizes one has done it is the "moment." And then, it passes. Lars Svendson in A Philosophy of Boredom *writes, "…the Moment is always indefinitely postponed. The Moment—the actual Meaning of life—only appears in a negative form that of absence, and the small moments (in love, art, intoxication) never last long."*

A place to sleep, Northern Thailand, October 13

The road out of Nong Hin is hemmed by rice paddies and I coast on its smooth surface immersed in an expansive silence. I try to hold myself in the moment. There have been days like this before, and more will follow. Days when I don't want to ride. After three quarters of an hour, we pull over at a gas station and buy a couple of yogurt drinks. I sense we are approaching something, a small town or national highway. This little corner store feels like a last stop, but last stop before what—entering a freeway or riding into nothing?

We chat at a picnic table with the girl, maybe fifteen, whose family owns the store and gas stand. At first, she kept her distance. Reticence, perhaps, shyness. For a few minutes she watched us sitting in the shade, then she smiled. Finally she joined us. I gesture at the map and point down the road, but she has no idea if there are any guesthouses. Two guys on a moped stop for gas and give us directions, nodding the whole time to our questions. They say there might be a hotel in three kilometres. By this time, it is after three o'clock. We have been stopping frequently to look forlornly at our bikes and surroundings. Our lack of enthusiasm is beginning to show.

"Are you ready to go?" I ask Rupert, who says yes then gazes off into space again.

We are so ready for an afternoon by an out-of-the-way waterfall. We had planned to ride fifty kilometres yesterday, but the town we were aiming for didn't appeal and the cool waterfall-fed pool I was hoping to swim in evaded us. We never saw a sign. I even went back a kilometer up-hill to look. Instead of an afternoon spent swimming, we spent it napping in an overly-warm guesthouse followed by another dinner of rice and vegetables.

With a long sigh—the kind dogs make, the kind kids make on slow summer days—we wave goodbye to the girl and two guys, remount our bikes and continue down the road. Only three more kilometers, we think, not far now.

After another five kilometers we stop at a convenience store. Behind it a few houses sit scattered on the slope. Maybe a small village, I think. A woman with grey hair and a cane points from her front porch across and up the road when we ask, in unison, our hands together, heads resting on them as one would pillows, about a guesthouse.

We follow a white pebble trail that cuts up behind a cluster of houses, then winds between trees and widens to a long gravel driveway. We turn left and see a gaggle of boys and girls playing volleyball in front of the makings of a temple. They freeze as we come into sight. Our eyes wander, taking in the dirt ground, the small huts lined behind the kids ahead of us and a large common house to the right in the distance. Three monks sit on a raised platform in the shade. Rupert takes off his helmet. He is wearing a long-sleeved cotton shirt, the same one he has worn for a few weeks to protect his skin from the sun. The children start to move again, excitedly, as if the King of Thailand has just walked up their path to greet them.

I keep my distance, not wanting to intrude, the only woman. As usual the monks are curious but seem content to observe me from a distance. Even the children stay away. Most young monks enter temples for a year or two but these men must be more dedicated because they are older than novices. Perhaps they have chosen a quiet half-built temple surrounded by hills in which to follow enlightenment and Buddhism. Standing on display, I am glad for the discretion of my loose shorts and shirt.

Rupert approaches, then gestures and points, nods, talks, then nods again and comes back to me. "We can stay here," he says, pointing at a tin-roofed hut just behind the group of kids. It looks about eight feet square and stands on thin stilts. Ours is a distance from the three others like it.

Rupert walks back to ask where we can bathe, while I walk my bike to the hut.

The children still haven't re-started their game. I feel their eyes on me and my bike as I lock it up, heave my bags up the rickety step ladder and toss them on the floor. I can just stand under the small covered patio, my head almost touching the rafters. Rupert will have to sit if he wants to enjoy the balcony view.

"There is a river, or something, just behind those trees further along the path we came up. We can bathe there," he says as he locks up his bike and passes me his bags. We get sarongs, towels, shampoo, and a change of clothes and head off to the "river".

By this time all the children have disappeared.

We walk along the trail we came in on and continue up the main road behind the compound. While Rupert was talking to the monks, I removed my padded shorts, thinking I could bathe in my loose nylon shorts and sports bra, the children on my mind. Now, while I am washing my cycling clothes in the river, the boys appear, strip down to their underwear, make a few gestures with their middle fingers followed by small fists pumping near their crotches and jump into the water. After splashing around and staring, they get out and walk further upstream. Without saying anything, Rupert and I gather our things and move a couple of meters in the opposite direction.

In faded shorts and a sport bra I bathe. The water comes up to my thighs, Rupert's shins. Our bellies and upper arms are pale, our legs and forearms the brown of the river. We know the children are nearby; there is no way they will pass up the chance to observe two crazy *farangs* bathing. But we pretend we are alone, throw socks at each other and swim around in the shallow water, the long day fading. It may not be a waterfall pool or the cleanest river, in fact is most likely irrigation pools for the nearby fields, but the water washes off the crystallized sweat and tired dirt. It washes off the ennui that has ridden my tail all day. I would like to stay in the warm shallow water, but the children's voices approach again.

By the time we get out, the girls have found us. Five of them, aged about three to nine, walk back to the compound with us, chatting all the way. One girl keeps asking questions and trying to tell me something. There was a storm and the river overflowed? No. There was a drought, the river dried up? No. Two children drowned in the irrigation pools while their mother did laundry nearby, their bodies swept away. This girl was one of the children, she nearly drowned? Noting her slightly wonky eyes, her slower steps, I keep nodding as she holds my hand trying to make me understand. Eventually, I stop worrying about what she is saying. I tell her about our adventures: the elephant taxis we saw when we first crossed into Thailand, the rain, and the sporadic mountain passes. She smiles, says a few more words and runs off with her friends. Just as I was starting to understand her, she is gone.

Later, after we wander the quiet main street with its dark scattered houses, a novice monk brings a mosquito net and a few blankets. We are grateful for the extra padding. He leaves and an older monk approaches who seems to want to connect, as we often do, wants to try his English and share his life. We listen, his words halting but direct and eager. Though not always clear, he is open and full of longing to share. Rupert listens encouragingly and asks a few questions about the area, while the man speaks of the temple that will soon stand in the spot where the cement pad sits, at the centre of the circle of huts. Before turning back toward the dark, the monk shakes Rupert's hand. We sit on our small deck, legs hanging off the edge, under the rail. I feel the world shrink to a single moment, to the open sky and the small light we cast surrounded by open unfaltering darkness. It is mid-October, but this close to the equator, every night, year-round at six in the evening, the sun drops, plop, and shuts down the light.

Inside we light our mosquito coils before spreading out the blankets and sliding under our sarongs. We carry no sleeping gear but use our large sarongs for blankets and stuff-sacks full of clothes for pillows. The floor is hard, but the blankets make it bearable. I dose off quickly, but am abruptly awoken by a chorus of sound. Sitting up, I realize the clatter of sound is rain on the tin roof. We both lie awake listening to the rain batter the corrugated tin so violently it sounds like the world coming to an end. I get up and peer out into the dark night expecting to see something, perhaps the monks and children standing in a circle outside watching us, but nothing moves except the fast running water that has formed a river around our bikes. I consider going out to move them, but decide not to. Instead, step into the rain and tip my head and let it wash my stinging eyes. Allergies or too much sun, I think, before turning back to bed.

Rupert shines his bike light on me, "Your eyes look terrible, he says. "Red and puffy." We crawl back under the mosquito net, shift and turn and fall back asleep.

Sugar Ride is about blood sugars and it is about the bicycles. Sometimes I am in front and the road is a vast river I glide down while Rupert rides my slipstream. Sometimes he rides hard to catch up or pass so I can coast in his draft. Then we slow, ride side-by-side, enter traffic, a stop light, mopeds and other bikes sidle up. Or, still in the zone we whiz past others on their bikes and have to break hard to stop when we spot a café. When someone waves or we think we should stop at the market, get duct tape, peanuts, bread, a bottle of shampoo or menstrual pads, Band-Aids.

Ninh Binh-ish, Vietnam, September 13

"Hey, where you going?" A guy on a moped pulls alongside me.

"Just up the street."

"You need a hotel?" He is riding in a pack with other motorcyclists.

"No, I don't think so."

"You want to go on a trek?"

"Uh, no I'm okay. Thanks." I try to ride away, avoiding eye-contact but before he will let me go, he hands me a business card—*Cycling Adventures in Vietnam*—I shove it in my pocket and laugh. "Can't he see we're doing that?!" I say to Rupert who rolls up beside me.

"Crazy," he agrees as we slowly pedal into the town looking around as we go.

In a room in a downtown hotel. There is that body of water. That totem pole, jogger, black-nosed dog. This driftwood sculpture, that water-side brewpub. The trickle of drain water and the excitement of sparrows. I am walking these paths away from home. I am home. I see how creating and destructing go hand in hand. How I can carry the weight of grief, the weight of the world in my thoughts, and I can carry the child-joy of the bike ride. I am in a room. I am on Lekwungen territory. I am on my bike. I am in another country.

Off the Highway near Ninh Binh, Vietnam, September 13

"Think of bicycles as ride-able art that can just about save the world."
—Grant Petersen

With a hand drawn map from an adventure café in town, we ready to leave the main road and explore a bit of the back country.

We find a gravel trail, but unsure, stop to consult the map. Rupert leans over and asks a man who is pushing his moped back toward the road. He smiles a toothless grin and shakes his head, waving rough bent fingers up a bit further to the next road.

A gaggle of women and chickens mark our muddy pock-marked path. As expected, the road is rough. We follow it through a collection of houses built from wood and cement now moss-green or dirt-brown. I smile, shyly, wanting to appear friendly, not as sure of myself as I was back on the road with the swarm of young men on mopeds.

We pass small wood shacks with chickens running about and pigs snorting in the background. The houses sit low to the ground. Mud has seeped up from the ground around the lower seams where outside walls meet ground. Women stop mid-sweep to watch us. I smile but keep pedaling. It is our second day out of Hanoi, and we ride side-by-side for the first time.

We round a corner and see a group of five children. At first, I think they are just playing in the road but then I realize, by their stern faces, that they plan to stop us. The tallest girl, with long brown hair, wears a red t-shirt and a serious expression. We make furtive eye-contact and keep going, slowly and steadily on the rough dirt road. The bright blue rain covers on our panniers not only protect the material from sun and the contents from rain, they also hide the openings and extra food and water we've shoved in at the last minute. They look like seamless, bulbous bags with no obvious openings. I fix my eyes on the oldest girl. As we get closer, the children begin to run ahead of us. Then, as we catch up, they grab our back racks or panniers. I nearly fall, nearly stop.

"Keep pedaling!" Rupert yells.

Panic hits me followed by a sense of the ridiculous—maybe they just want to play. There is nothing fun in any of this—the tall girl's stern look, her and the other children holding onto my pannier, and my fear that I will topple on one of them or hit a rock and bend my wheel. My fear that we are being stupid. Ahead, Rupert has broken free of his hanger-on, but mine, the tall strong girl, persists. She runs alongside me, her hand gripping my pannier. It seems she will hold on forever.

Perhaps a grandmother yells at her, perhaps a mother, or perhaps she just gets tired. Perhaps she stepped on a rock or lost one of her flip-flops. Perhaps her friends are now too far away and she feels vulnerable, the last still holding on. I don't know, but she lets go.

I urge my bulky bike up the rocky hill, my heart racing. I pedal and wobble over potholes and through mud ditches. I pick up speed downhill then hit mud and another cluster of potholes. The bones in my body clang and crash against each other. My hands are white with gripping, my ass throbs from the sharp contact with the seat. I lurch to a stop and put my foot down beside Rupert who waits just around the corner.

"Huh," I say and he looks back to where we've come from.

"That was weird," he says.

I wonder what they had planned for us. Had they hoped for money, cameras, bikes or trinkets? I can't think what we have of value to a group of children. And yet everything must be of value to them. Maybe it's just our difference, maybe just a game or maybe anything we have or do is just more interesting than what they have or were doing moments before.

"Weird," I say again.

"Who knows," Rupert says, "who knows what kids will do. They were a wild little tribe though."

I love Rupert's easy summary. I love how he doesn't question his own motives in riding as fast as he could, love that he trusts the action of fleeing from a wild little tribe. "Well, I hope these inland cliffs are worth it," I say, my frustration seeping out in my bitter tone.

Somewhere along the road from Hanoi to Danang or from young to middle aged, things began to get serious. Somewhere we stopped laughing. Somewhere we let our heads fall back and the laughter spilled. Somewhere we danced too, made love the first time again. Personal grief split us open; the grief of the world. Everywhere there were beggars. Some would find us, some watch, some grab our bikes. Beggars or just wild kids, we were never sure. Bicycles and bodies; crank, shaft, lungs, legs.

We continue on the rough road toward the cliffs. My bones rattle and my sit-bones, the pointy bones in my ass, scream. We plummet fast, down and down, and all I can think of is the ride back up. Over the sound of my bike bouncing and my bones rattling, I can hear the trickle of water as we pass through a small forest. The trail opens to a gravel road with a parking lot to the right and ahead and to the left, near a river-side ledge, a small white house. The house is a café, an English country villa, with a shaded patio surrounded by impatiens, plumeria and orchids. We have stumbled onto a luxury restaurant for visitors, mostly French, who have come to explore the old colony, to make contact with long ago family, a father or uncle stationed here before the war.

We walk our bikes, letting them almost fall down a set of long, low steps, then lean them in a corner and wait to be pointed to a seat. The tables have white cloths, proper napkins and tall water glasses. The menu is all Vietnamese fodder, but catered to the tourist, so Rupert finally gets his spring rolls. I feel a mild sense of culture shock. Looking around, I flatten down my bandana and rub the dust off my cheeks. The maître d' hands us each a cool wet towel to wipe our hands. We also wipe our faces and necks. The mere sight of our dusty, sweaty bodies delights one woman, sitting nearby in pale pinks and whites. She's originally from England.

"Where are you traveling from?" she asks in the Queens accent.

"We've ridden from Hanoi over a few days," Rupert says, adding details of our journey to the woman's excited little hand claps.

"My husband was here in the war. I'm living in France now."

We both nod, waiting for more.

"Have you been to see the cliffs?"

"Not yet," I reply this time.

She smiles warmly, then asks, "Are you Americans?"

"No, we're from the west coast of Canada."

"How delightful! I have a distant cousin in Hull, have you been to Quebec?"

The conversation continues in this way until our food arrives and the woman's tour group, having had their tea, heads off to visit the gift shops. "Ta-ra then," she says. "And do be careful."

After our utterly divine lunch, we decide to forgo the water tour and instead stick close to our bikes. Tall sharp cliffs meshed in by vibrant green rice stalks and soul-calming quiet enfold me as we cycle a narrow paved trail. The canal winds between the cliffs, under the path and on through green fields. How different one moment can be from the next, that tribe of bike-grabbing kids fading from my thoughts as I follow Rupert. Now I can hear my own breathing. I can hear the whirr of tires on the soft rocky path. I look up and up to rich green hills and vibrant blue sky. It's so easy to call this an adventure. Yet as days like this become our norm—kind, curious and helpful adults and ferocious children or frightened and puzzled adults and friendly children—it becomes easy to summarize the whole experience into the word adventure. Who said "the days are long but the years short"? I feel that. The weeks are short and the days are packed, detailed, exasperating, enlightening. Always the landscape offers a rich architecture: hills or rocky peaks, houses and cathedrals; walls decorated with Coke posters, communist-style anti-AIDs and one-child-per-family posters.

We follow the trail to a large gravel parking lot with a Chinese Buddhist temple at the back. Encased in leafy trees, its orange gate pokes out. "Strange to see something so familiar," Rupert whispers.

The sight of the orange gates dramatically whisks us back to Japan. They remind us of China's influence on Southeast Asia and Japan's influence here, as an occupier from 1940-1945.

"Not strange as in unexpected," I offer, and he agrees as he coasts ahead.

We follow a group of French tourists into the temple grounds. While the priest in his austere black cotton robe shows the carvings and where to drop coins for prayer, we examine the pillars at the front of the small temple—carved dragons entwine themselves around and around the pillar. I enter behind the last of the bus tour, and the priest gestures for money. His face is marvellously lined, his eyes full of mischief. I drop a few coins, the equivalent of a quarter, into a bowl. He grins, then hands me a candle. I walk over and light one, then pray, Japanese style—my hands together before my face, a slight bow—for a safe journey.

After the other tourists leave, the priest disappears behind the temple, perhaps into a small house at the back and changes into his white cotton trousers and shirt. He returns in his casual clothes and giggles while pointing out the bulging noses and eyes, the curling goatees on the dragons entwining themselves around the two pillars at the opening to the temple. He suddenly smiles and waves to Rupert to catch his attention. He points to a small table, inviting us to join him for tea.

After brewing the jasmine tea and pouring, he sits back and fans himself. Rupert decides to try some of the Chinese characters he learned in Japan. He scribbles on a scrap of paper. The priest understands, grinning now from ear to ear and nodding while Rupert sketches out the character for rain, wanting to know if the priest knows what weather lies ahead. The priest, taking his pen, sketches back. We drink tea and I quietly challenge my stomach to hold it all down—semi boiled water out of cold-water-washed cups.

Before we leave, I hand the priest a small Canada pin, but he won't take it. He gestures instead for me to pin it to his pocket. Then gestures again, he wants it in the centre. His eyes sparkle with mischief, while I move it and smile at him. I step back and bow, deeply, thanking him for his kindness, laughing eyes and friendly face.

A recent Globe and Mail *article explores where fear of the other comes from in white middle-class America: lack of exposure, "White people who live in areas where they're immersed in longstanding populations of immigrants and minorities—that is big cities—don't generally tend to vote for the politics of racial intolerance." Though we were in Asia, and I am not speaking of voting trends, it seems clear that exposure to the other makes the other seem less threatening. To the children who tried to stop us, perhaps we were a rare and scary phenomenon while to the priest we were unique but also familiar to his daily tour buses of visitors.*

Riding floodwaters to Hua Hin, Thailand, October 25

"Why can't a bicycle stand up by itself?
Because it's two tired."—Anon

Visibility is low with fog rolling in as we pedal away from the floating market on a narrow back-country road. At a bridge I stop to look back toward the market town and notice how quickly the water is rising. We have about twenty kilometres to ride before the next town. Tired, we bike through a tunnel of rain and fog. The wind pushes and the rain dispirits us. Fields to the left and right flood. We watch as distant buildings, some houses, some temples, gradually begin to float, the greenery vanishing.

At a covered gas station we huddle to eat, then continue. We stop again in a small town with little more than a market and bus station. We are just too wet. Saddled by rain, the day falling dark, we wonder if we have entered the throes of rainy season and if it will ever end. We want to look at the climate section of our *Lonely Planet*, but don't want to see how wet all our belongings are. The rain covers on our panniers won't keep the rain from getting in the back and through the seams. After two hours a bus finally comes. It isn't air conditioned, thank goodness.

We lug our bikes through the door, push them down the aisle to the back and sit caged in by them. Rupert shivers so I dig around in his bag, which presses up against my left shin, and pass him a sweater. I seem to have both back ends, so find mine next.

Outside, the rain keeps falling. Due to flooded streets the bus has to bypass a small town and detour onto a larger road. The bus assistant comes back, now and then, to report on the road conditions.

I lift my head from my bike rack as the bus jerks to a stop. The assistant comes toward us: "Here is Phetburi. You get off and wait." She helps pull out our bikes, and the bus disappears. We stand with our feet in water, water almost up to my knees and Rupert's mid-calf.

"This is why they have such high sidewalks," I say, stepping up.

We aren't sure if we should just wait where we are, but urge our slippery heavy bikes up the sidewalk under an awning and wait.

"I need to pee."

"What if the bus comes?"

"I can't wait. Look at me, I'm soaked. The rain is making it worse. I'll just go down that way and ask." I point to the left to some shops. "I'll be quick." I run down a few doors, pop my head in the first shop. No one's there. At the second shop, a woman smiles at me, "Hawng suam?"

She nods and leads me down the back of her narrow shop and points into a room. A squat toilet, raised on a platform with a large well-like cistern greets me. "Thank goodness," I think, as I peel my wet shorts and paddies off and hover. Then, I began to get the tooth-chattering giggles. "Oh, no paper." I never thought to look before starting. I have to be quick. I'm shivering. "Oh well, I'm so wet already," I say aloud to myself.

"Khap khun kaa," I say to the shop keeper, she looks up and nods, then passes me a bag of Chinese-style rice snacks. I bow and run back to Rupert standing with his arms crossed to keep warm, shivering. Now he needs to go. I point the way, while snacking on the spicy crackers.

I begin to wonder if a bus will actually come. If we were home, and this were a snowstorm of equal severity, all business would stop. Trucks filled with people and couples on mopeds pass, their wheels half-buried in water. I imagine we will become part-fish, a shiver goose-bumping my skin.

Finally, the bus comes. As we drag our bikes on board, four cockroaches take refuge on my left leg. They scamper up out of the water, run along my shin and onto the raised sidewalk. I freeze. Rupert catches my eye as a shiver goes from my toes to the top of my head. I can see he is trying to have as little reaction as possible but almost imperceptibly shrugs.

"Waaaaa," I say shuddering.

The bus assistant is happy to welcome us on board. He pockets our 100 bhat, a considerable sum, but we do have bikes, and he no doubt has a family to feed. Weary, we rest our heads on the seat back or pannier pressed into us and sleep for the hundred and thirty kilometers to Hua Hun.

I wake as the bus pulls into a city. Rain continues to cascade out from the bus's back wheels, spraying fountains of water up into the dim light of evening. We stand under a small shelter and look at our maps trying to figure out where we are. We need to locate a guesthouse. A group of young guys on mopeds watches us until finally one comes over and offers to lead us to a good place.

"Okay," we say in unison, too tired to contemplate the risks of anything beyond being wet.

He leads us off the main road along flooded back streets toward the ocean. We then cut to the left, taking a narrow lane adjacent to a fancy hotel. Through the fog of rain I think I see trees shaped like animals. For once, I'm not seeing things. I spot a giant rooster, a giraffe and my second snake of the day. I should be paying attention but am mesmerized by the topiary and the haze of rain. The animal trees seem to follow as we pass.

The moped driver's wheels spin out for a moment before he lurches and continues down another alley. I follow, my feet dunking in water with each spin of my pedals, my wheels sending out fans of water behind and in front, hitting my face. Then something stops me. My front wheel is blocked. For a moment, I freeze, puzzled, my wheels unmoving. Then my bike topples and I land, feet still on pedals, in the water. I jump to my feet just as Rupert catches up.

"I-I-I think there is a lip there or a curb of some sort," I say, shivering as I point down to where my bike has drowned. I lift it up, lean it against me, then try to pull my padded shorts away from my crotch and ring them out. They are soaked to my skin and I need to pee again. Our moped guide comes back.

"Okay?"

"Yes, here we come!" I answer in a cheery sing-song voice.

Rupert stands and lifts his front wheel over the curb and carries on.

Sitting is torture, the wet shorts mush up against my crotch so that a violent shiver runs through me. I am desperate to get out of them. I follow until we coast down a narrow shopping street that ends at the Mod Guest House. Seen through the rain the sign looks like it says *My God*.

"You like this place, very good," says our friend who shakes our hands, bows and drives off. I stand with our bikes in the rain while Rupert walks down the ramp to the entrance.

"Yup, looks good," he says returning to pull me out of a crowd that has gathered in fascination. I imagine I look like a cat that has been yanked by its fur out of a bathtub.

The minute we are in the room, I leave Rupert to lock up bikes and throw myself into the bathroom, stripping off wet clothes as I go. I can't believe I am now going to have a cold shower. My feet and hands are prunes; even my knees are wrinkled. My only thought: will I have dry clothes to put on as the grit and sand of the day rinses down the drain at my feet.

Mod Guest house had stilts that stood it out over the ocean. As we slept we could hear the lapping tide. Everything we owned was wet unless it was in a bag. Our passports, money, letters in varying languages explaining the drugs and tickets home were in Ziploc bags under our clothes. They too were wet at the edges. Our bikes were our horses, we were nomads in a wild world. It was a gift to be helped. We leapt at friendships, then shied away. We wrapped a protective shield around each other. This is how we survived. This is being without a home. Finding a home in each other—our chilly damp bodies keeping each other warm.

I want to say to my younger self—take note. Look up. Are you paying attention? Are you enjoying this? Enjoy it. Look around, I want to say. Get out of your head.

Alor Setar, Malaysia, November 7

We exit the toll road and enter the chaos of suburban streets stretching long fingers toward the city centre. As in other Asian cities, the buildings here are low, only one or two stories. Though they are the familiar crumbling colonial buildings we've been passing for months, the wide and well-kept road tells us we are in the wealthiest country thus far. There are even freshly painted dividing lines and arrows on the asphalt. As we ride closer to the centre of town the mini strip malls are gradually replaced by the crumbling buildings of old town. We quickly find cheap lodging at Yuan Fang Hotel. Eighteen ringgit with shared bathroom. Rupert immediately brightens. The walls of our room don't reach the ceiling, for ventilation, and the window looks over a busy street, but suddenly we feel like we've arrived in Malaysia.

Once checked in, we head off to explore the streets and old buildings. "Malaysia is a kingdom of Sultans," I say as we walk, reading to Rupert from our squashed and bedraggled *Lonely Planet*. "Did you know, 'Kedah is the only state that still holds the remnants of Hindu Kingdoms of the eighth and ninth century?' In fact, the current royal family can trace its line back to Hindu times. It says here that 'The British placed restrictions on the sultans during colonialism, much to the Malays' opposition. On August 30, 1957 Malaysia was granted independence and the sovereign rights of the rulers were guaranteed in the constitution.'" We reach the museum, which was once the Royal Palace or the Big Hall. Inside we face wall after wall of royal paintings. I look at a few paintings, then go back to the *Lonely Planet*'s descriptions of Malaysia's history, read something on a wall, then slump back hoping we aren't going to have to read every single inscription on every inch of the museum. I actually prefer learning about the country from the road and the seat of my bike. I become mid-day-museum sluggish.

"Let's go," I say and Rupert finally agrees.

Out in the hot sun we circle the round white building and then walk, hand in hand, back toward town. After so many weeks of following or being followed by the other, I find it strange and comforting to be walking side-by-side, within hearing of each other.

Back near our hotel, we note that Kentucky Fried Chicken represents the most obvious western import here. On account of the Islamic Malay and Hindu Indians, chicken is probably the easiest meat to agree on, Rupert and I decide, chatting as we walk. The colours of cloth from bright batiks hanging in shops next to silk saris and simple cotton robes tells more of the country's multiculturalism than the white-washed colonial buildings. The newspaper stand sells papers in Chinese, English, Malay and Tamil. As we walk along the busy street we become aware that the country is on holiday. Deepavali, we learn. Though some shops are open for business, they all seem to be Chinese-owned. Wandering around looking for a bank to exchange our yen traveller's cheques for ringgit, we stumble upon a movie theatre.

"Oh." I say, excitedly. After a close inspection of the movie listings we discover that *The Thomas Crown Affair* is playing, staring Pierce Brosnan. We've not heard of it but it sounds intriguing. Besides, we've not been out to a movie in over four months. Nor have we watched TV or heard English on the radio. In addition to this one western film there is an array of Indian films. "We really should see an Indian film," I say. "Apparently they are a riot of audience participation."

"Hmmm," Rupert agrees, inspecting Pierce Brosnan's movie. The pull of escape, to slip completely away from our daily travel grind and into familiar but alien world, hooks us both.

The Thomas Crown Affair is a remake of the 1968 movie starring Steve McQueen and Faye Dunaway. Dunaway appears in the remake as Crown's psychologist. Crown is a wealthy bored financier who steals a Monet from the MoMA; Catherine Banting, played by Rene Russo, is the insurance agency's bounty hunter.

After two and a half months of cycling in Southeast Asia I sit in the movie theatre in Alor Setar mesmerised by the familiarity of what I see on the screen: the city streets and comforts, the stunning house and wealth. I am overwhelmed by Russo's clothes (I have one pair of rayon pants and two t-shirts). I am astounded and swept off the earth listening to the actors speak English, the speed of it. No longer in Asia, I am in the movie's world. I almost weep watching this world that, truthfully, is utterly alien to me, but which seems familiar because everyone in there speaks English. Because Western art in the MoMA, because taxi cabs and cool lace-up boots. Have I looked in a mirror recently? Do I know I am muscled and paired down to legs for cycling and arms for cycling and blonde hair and freckles? No. None of that matters. I no longer think of my body as an object. In the world of the movie, the body, the clothes and the objects of wealth all matter and all of them come so easy.

Outside the movie, I pay attention to my body as machine with its varying quirks and pains. With its rising and falling blood sugar levels. I know I have an ass because it aches much of the time. The rest of my body is reduced to eating, drinking, testing, taking insulin, and riding. Our showers are cold, our days long and hot and utterly free. But in the theatre, I want popcorn, want to hold my husband's hand and vanish into that other world up on the screen.

The other night, I re-watched The Thomas Crown Affair. *The thing I long for now, other than Russo's clothing, (some things just don't change) is the glider that lands them in a far flung field of cows, the cell in his pocket, the private jet, the flight to the Caribbean, the house in the sunny warm Caribbean, her enthusiastic response to architecture, churches, cliffs as they drive up through forest to his mountain top villa. But their freedom seems too easy, and clichéd.*

What I want is the adventure. Not carefree but free of the worries of aging parents and a growing kid. I want to be out on the road on my bike again, the wind at my back, some song overplaying in my head, my body working hard for every mile. I want to see teak houses and hear children laughing and connect to the world even if it means struggling, but struggling in a larger context than body, house, street, car, city.

After the movie, Rupert and I walk because I am too worked up to sleep. The streets of Alor Setar are quiet and we are nervous about where we are and where we have to go. The only white faces for over a hundred kilometres, until we reach Georgetown, we stand out and we don't know what that means on our second day in Malaysia. We learn country by country or city by city on this trip what it means. So, our walk is short and that night I sleep badly. The short walls of our room do not block out the sounds of snoring and hacking and partying. Revved up on the movie and surrounded by men's snorting and spitting I am up and in the shower with the rooster's crow at five.

Some moments fade into the recesses so that all that is left is a feeling, or a sense of something forgotten, ghost memories pentimento between the lines. We nearly turned around after our first day in Malaysia and went back to Thailand. The price difference almost too much. In three months we saw two movies, we went to one play, saw several dance performances, ate flying morning glory where the cooked greens were thrown by the chef from atop the cookhouse roof and caught by the waiter (passing through swarms of mosquitos on their way).

First day of Conjunctivitis, Thailand, October 14

I wake to sunlight, the chatter of children and the realization that I can't open my eyes. My hands fumble over lids coated in salt and sand thick as mortar. With my thumb and index finger I pry my eyes open, then gently scrape a nail over the top and bottom lashes to clean them. I blink a few times but cannot focus. My eyes sting.

"They don't look good," Rupert says peering at me.

Yellow mucus begins to cake and dry if I don't continuously blink. We pack and eat stale bread with peanut butter on the low porch. I run water over my eyes again, dab at them with the corner of my t-shirt and get ready to go. The children are gone, but a few of the monks wave, from a distance, to me. Rupert walks over to return the blankets and give our thanks. He is patted on the back, I can see him shaking hands in thanks. We both bow deeply before riding off.

I follow a bike-length behind Rupert down the trail and onto the road. I squint and moan. All I can see is the steep incline of road ahead of my yellow-shirted husband. I follow the retro-reflective white strip on Rupert's pannier covers. Through slit eyes, I check our progress. From the top of the first hill, we stop to look out at the scenery and so Rupert can check my puffy, mucus-weeping eyes. The sunlight stings but we have eighty kilometers to ride before the next town so I have do my best to ignore them. The scene before us strikes me as both beautiful and terrible at the same time.

"Why," I ask Rupert, "can't they build roads around the hills. Every single one crests over the top."

I am in a sour mood, feeling sorry for myself. My eyes seep and ache, pus gums my lids together so I stop and squirt water over them again and again. The wind is agony and my bike's not gearing well; when I drop to a low gear for a hill, then up to a high one to go down the hill, I can't get it back down when the next hill comes along. Everything is wearing out. We barely speak. Rupert knows how miserable I am, can hear me grunting and cursing behind him. Tears help soothe my eyes.

I hate pushing my bike up hills. Even if my legs and chest ache and it is hard and slow I'd rather ride. Pushing means negotiating the swinging front wheel and the off-balance and weighted back. Pushing means lugging, means giving in to the hill. Pushing means being like Sisyphus, his awkward clumsy rock my machine, it means fighting both the road and my mood. Nonetheless, completely at my wits end with the gears, I walk up-hill. This floods me with an unalterable sense of utter failure. The futility of dragging my bike, weighed down, straight up, is also exhausting.

Plantain trees line the road. Their long broad leaves shade the shoulder and the small green fingers of fruit stick out in handfuls. I entertain the fantasy of a bus, one that doesn't take bikes, one that would force me to leave my bicycle behind and quickly get to a guesthouse with a cold shower I could stand under all afternoon, to soothe my eyes and weary body. Or if I still had my bike, I'd leave it outside the guesthouse. With any luck, it might be stolen.

I get back on my bike at the top and coast down the fourth hill, then start pedaling as the fifth hill climbs steeper. At this point, my bike really turns on me. The chain and gears lock. I can't drop from third to second and the chain derails, the pedals seize. I curse and roll to a stop. I huff and puff in hot fast breaths as my eyes begin to tear up. I drop my bike, kick it and walk away. This is the bike I brought with me from Canada to Japan. My baby. My love.

Rupert leaves his bike and walks down toward me. He smiles and tilts his head; we say nothing. He gets on my bike, knees almost hitting his chin, and rides, stopping to make adjustments to the derailleur so the chain will drop down or up into higher and lower gears as needed. I walk his bike up the rest of the hill. At the top, I plop down on a bench in a pull-out area, semi-shaded, a kind of open-air, cement bus shelter. Rupert adjusts the gears some more and greases the chains while I sit with eyes closed. The bike, hills, my eyes have thoroughly defeated me. Off in the distance, more hills. More winding roads and no bus or fantasy jet to pick me up and take me away from this misery.

Behind us, a waterfall crests down a hill, then turns to a river running all the way back to the village we've spent the morning riding away from. "It's beautiful," I finally say to Rupert who is finishing with the chain grease. He comes and sits beside me and I lean my chin on his shoulder and look out beyond.

"I can't believe how high we've climbed," he says.

I nod, thinking how all day I've been riding to get the hills over with. My eyes throb and tear up.

As I get ready to set off toward the sixth hill, Rupert pulls a bunch of plantains off a nearby branch. The fruit is sweet and sticky and while I eat I realize how desperately I need it. Low blood sugars are adding to my sense of utter misery, my sluggish, weak legs and weepy eyes. With a deep sigh, I swing my leg back over my bike ready to attempt living in the moment of each hill. I try not to fight, gear down a little earlier, and rather than thinking "when I get to the top I'll be done" I just pedal and breathe. My blurry teary eyes help. I can't really see how steep the hill is so I stop trying to. When the wind comes, I try to believe it is helping. I chant, "This ain't no heartbreak hill," until that chant becomes Cher's "Do you believe in life after love?"

I wonder what Rupert's definition of love and endurance is? Maybe this: having the tools and knowing how to use them.

Ho Chi Minh Trail, Vietnam, September 16

Ho Chi Minh Trail
0 kilometers
1970–

We stop in front of the sign, surprised. We are at the beginning of the road used by the Vietnamese to transport people, weapons and food during the war. I am dumbstruck. "Are we really standing here, in one of the most heavily bombed areas in the world?" I say.

Rupert shrugs his shoulders and looks around. After nearly twenty-five years since the war, ruined land surrounds us. Rice fields that look more like pot holes with only a few stalks of rice growing in them. It takes a few minutes to absorb not only the landscape but the history wrapped up in the name of this trail. The Vietcong used the Ho Chi Minh trail because it was in a heavily forested area. Now it is a barren landscape as far as the eye can see. The legacy of Agent Orange. No trees. No birdsong. As we look around, Rupert points out the lines of craters from the B52's bombing runs. As the bombs fell, hard bedrock was flung up onto fertile soil.

We ride the Ho Chi Minh through small villages. In some sections we gingerly pedal over crops of grain spread across the trail to dry in the sun. We are almost at Dong Loc—the village with a war memorial marked on our map. We ride up hill on loose gravel anticipating the town we feel certain we are coming to. Small houses begin to line the street that opens to a T-junction. At the intersection the road continues up toward more houses, or sweeps down and to the left. We follow it down toward a huge white statue of human figures, their arms raised to the sun. Behind the statue the road ends at a building, the war museum.

We stop in front of the statue, quickly realizing this place is more village than town, more memorial and museum than village. A small group of men and children have followed us from the intersection down to the base of the statue. As we sit on its steps and pull out lunch—crackers, stale bread and peanut butter—the men and children gather around us, nodding as one or two men occasionally point to the museum and say a few words. I quickly give myself my lunch time insulin, pulling out the pen, twisting the needle in and administering insulin while Rupert distracts the curious crowd.

As we are packing up, a young man on a moped approaches the quiet, watching crowd and asks the typical first question: "Where are you from?"

As we chat about where we live and the Vietnam War, the man, Lee, explains the statue's meaning. It represents the victory of the Vietnamese as well as friendship, since it was built by Vietnamese and American vets—Americans who came here to find their lost family and friends.

The men around us nod, knowingly. They are all in their fifties, or older, and add to the story so that Lee is speaking Vietnamese and English almost in unison. As we chat, ominous clouds roll across the sky. On Lee's advice, we move to the memorial museum and put our bikes under cover to wait out the rain. We wave to the crowd quickly dispersing to escape the oncoming rain.

The museum is an L-shaped building. The entrance is in the smaller part, which contains a kitchen and what looks like living quarters. Down the long left arm of the building, one wall boasts floor to ceiling windows, while the opposite holds a display of black and white photographs of American and Vietnamese veterans standing in ditches or by airplanes. Each step we take echoes on the hard floors, reverberating off the constant thrum of rain. Lee walks behind us, or stands near Rupert to talk. He isn't reticent with me and answers our questions easily.

Rain and thick grey fog has enveloped the village and museum; we feel truly encased in the black and white images as the world beyond them is drained of colour too. The clouds and rain turn the sky an iridescent grey which reflects onto the trees. The green hills and ground are alight with water and reflected light. The rain comes down hard and loud and I stand breathless in the shelter of the museum.

Lee, our second friend of the day after Viet Ha and her family, works in a church. His moped is piled with books, all religious and educational texts. As we talk we all realize he's not covered them. He was too concerned with helping get our bikes out of the rain. The three of us run out to cover the now damp books precariously balanced on his bike.

The museum is actually only one room out of the large complex, which houses photographs of soldiers who fought in the area. It also shows pictures of several American GIs. Many still return to find lost friends, to connect with those experiences from their youth and come to some kind of understanding of what it meant to fight here. Perhaps they come to find peace.

Six people live in the building, maybe caretakers or Vietnamese veterans. I ask Lee if many Vietnamese visit.

"No," he says. "It is too far out of the way and there are no paved roads."

But when the rain stops, and we are readying to leave, a nice car pulls up and a middle-class Vietnamese family of four spills out. They could be American.

When we lived in Japan we were in a community of expats. British, American, Canadian, Australian and New Zealanders lived in our city or nearby. We were simplified down to a small group of Caucasians, though we weren't all Caucasian. One American was Philippine, one was African-American. I guess we were Anglo-Canadians. To the Japanese, on some level, we were all the same. To us too. Over time. Let's say I was taking the train to Kitakyushu

and from the train I saw a petit though slightly overweight woman with blond hair. I would immediately categorize her as a single person—Sarah. She might not be Sarah, but she had Sarah hair and build. My Caucasian or Foreign reading simplified, but my Asian reading became more refined. I could tell if someone was Korean or Japanese, even if the Korean person hid it by taking a Japanese name. I could tell if someone would be open to meeting us, or not. Could tell if a person I was approaching would begin to back away, or pretend to not hear me, or smile and move toward me. If they would hear that I was speaking Japanese or instantly say they didn't speak English. To the Japanese, we were easy to pick out. Rupert, my sister and I cycled to Hagi over a couple of days. In one town, my sister and I left Rupert with our bikes and walked to a small store to buy snacks. When we walked in, the woman there said, "Where is the tall man with you?"

Dong Loc to Ha Tinh, Vietnam, September 16

"The rain has stopped," Lee says. "Let's go."

We follow him around the museum, our wheels spinning, spraying thick red mud. According to Lee, we are only twenty kilometers from Ha Tinh. Because of the rain we must contend with slippery mud instead of gravel.

At a gully where locals are laying gravel to raise the road, we have to cross on a fifteen centimeter-wide cement ledge. Lee goes first and Rupert follows. They both carefully balance their wheels on the narrow ledge to cross. I lift my front wheel up and hoist the heavy back and begin to pedal in a low gear. On my right: thick grey mud, the same mud that coats my legs and backs of my panniers. To my left: a deep pool of water. I use toe-cages to hold my feet on the pedals but have taken my right foot out. I want to be ready to drop my foot into the mud if I lose my balance. As I slowly pedal I try to focus on going straight, but once my mind hooks onto the possibility of falling...I fall, bike and body into the mud, but not the pool. My right leg catches on my sprockets as I go down. I quickly stand up, just fast enough to save my bike from sinking fully into the wet ooze. Lee jumps off his bike and comes back to roll mine out. Two of the work men run toward me. No chance pretending I am fine. Some of the women workers look and point at my bleeding knee with concerned expressions. Rupert stays where he is, as if catching an impromptu fringe performance. He watches my rescuers surround and buoy me up.

One workwoman offers bandages and a tissue. The tissue works better as it sticks to my damp skin, but my rescuers insist on the bandage. I tuck the tissue in my pocket, push the bandage over the cut and bow my thanks. A few of my saviours pat me on the back. Lee and one of the other men help to clear the muck off my bike as I walk alongside them feeling useless. When Lee holds my bike out to me, I swing a leg over. Already in low gear, I stand on the pedals and try to get the wheels to grab the road. Mud sprays out behind me as I begin my ascent.

I fall, everyone rushes to me. You have gathered by now that if anyone is going to fall it will be me. Just as well, I think. If it had been Rupert who would have come? In the movie version of Cheryl Strayed's Wild *a forest ranger brings her coffee in the morning, but none for the men she's camped with. He says she can get more when she's finished and then walks away, nodding at the men. It is a hilarious moment. In South East Asia there are huge benefits to being Rupert. But, because he is very tall, he has to cool his energy to not be misunderstood. To remain easy with men, and not too forward with women. Probably no one would rush to save him, except me.*

I rest my bike on its side while Rupert and I squat to look at it. He spins and I watch as the rear wheel picks up speed, then rubs against the brake, and stops. He spins again and the same happens. The wheel moves in a kind of wave-like manner, smooth for a second, then stops. My rear wheel has warped from all the weight I have been carrying.

I look at Rupert and sing the familiar few words from a ditty we sang on a road trip to Mount Aso in Japan: "Who's got a big old butt? Oh yeah." Eight of us had crammed into an uncomfortable van and when quarters got too close, Wil, our friend from California, started singing these lines. They stuck.

"Oh yeah," Rupert chimes in.

In addition to the rear wheel, my gears continue to worsen—crunching and grinding before shifting. Rupert's bike has been hanging on by a thread since we turned the axel around. The time has come to find a proper bike shop, a bike shop with tools that work on our bikes, bikes more modern than most of the tough machines we see on the roads.

We tweak my back wheel as best we can—loosen the brakes, adjust a few of the spokes and carry on. We need a shop, but need to keep riding to get to one.

The smooth road sets a straight course. My legs spin and my mind wanders. Songs and images coast in and out of my thoughts. I wonder where my parents are at this moment and what my sister is up to. She is dating a guy I met last summer on a visit home, a guy I didn't like. Half the time I see the world I am riding through, the rest of the time my eyes turn inward, see pieces of the world I've already ridden. Sometimes, I wonder what our future will hold. Rupert and I have talked of going to New Zealand after Christmas but because we didn't take up the awesome offer of Thai Vegetarian cooking lessons in exchange for English lessons in Phitsanulok, I believe we will likely settle at home. With his teaching degree, we can go anywhere from Victoria to a small school in the Yukon. A friend from Japan got a job in Nunavut, her surroundings the polar opposite of these mountains and forests hemmed in by rice fields. When we first crossed the border into Thailand I thought the paddies were small, but now we are as far west as we will go until we hit the west coast of Malaysia, and the fields are oceans of green stalks. Two hundred kilometers to our west is Myanmar or Burma and four hundred kilometers south Bangkok.

The road winds until we hit a bridge, on the other side the town of Phichit. We cycle over the bridge and quickly find a guy sitting outside a shop surrounded by bikes, so I pull over. By now it is obvious my wheel has a problem; it squeaks as it rubs the brake and makes a wump-wump sound as I push the bike toward the shop entrance. I take off my panniers and roll the bike into the shop but the owner crosses his arms and shakes his head. After wrestling the panniers back on, we go further up the street. The second bike shop owner also shakes his head and laughs.

"You go that way," he says, stretching his arm to point down the street. My frustration wells.

"What's going on?" Rupert asks.

"Why won't any of these guys even touch my bike?"

Rupert shrugs, as uncommunicative as the shop owners. I'd so love to ride off into the sunset, away from all these annoying men but I am too hot and sticky. Besides, my ride, were it a horse, would be shot by now. It feels like we are in *The Good, The Bad and the Ugly* again, a movie where the locals stare at alien newcomers. *Oooo ooo ooo ooo ooo*, I would say, if I were in any mood to laugh.

We struggle to get my bags back on, deciding it best to find the police and ask about accommodation and a bike shop that might actually help.

We ride down the street passing near-closing shops. I spot a pharmacy, toy store and bookstore before the second bike shop owner catches up to us on his moped and stops in front of me. He motions for us to follow, leading the way to another bike shop, but it is closed. He then leads us to a small convenience store with a guesthouse upstairs. All we've seen so far in this town is a motel charging 500 bhat, but the elderly couple running this place charge only one hundred. We bow, graciously, to the bike shop guy and he smiles, the first smile we have seen in this town. I dig in my pannier and pass him a Canada pin. His smile deepens and spreads to his eyes. My irritation begins to fade while I sit with the bikes and Rupert runs upstairs to check out the room.

"Our own bathroom with a throne even," he says, running back down to meet me. I maneuver my panniers off my bike a third time and lug them up while he negotiates a place for the bikes. Home sweet home.

There is a lesson here about privilege. I had come, perhaps, to expect to get help having been given so much help. The privilege of being a white visible minority on a bike. A friendly unknown anomaly. Of course, not everyone wanted to help. Sometimes the very sight of us set off alarms because of the white skin and the likelihood of no language. Or alarms left by history. I expected these bike shop guys to stop what they were doing and help. Probably they took one look at the bike, being bike guys, and knew they were the wrong kind of experts. They were the wedge and hammer bike repair men and I needed the allen keys and wrenches guy.

Nakhon Sawan, Thailand, October 19

From the bed in our second-story room I can see the full moon through the window. I watch until what feels like a long blink and the moon is the sun and it is time get up again. In the night, small black bugs have settled over us, our clothes, panniers, towels, everything. We take a few minutes to shake them off, dress and head out the door to re-locate yesterday's bike shop.

We ride down a quiet dusty road. Not much is open at this early hour but thankfully the bike shop is. Tricycles surround the owner perched on the sidewalk tightening a bolt on a back wheel. My rear wheel is so obviously warped, the mechanic stands as I enter and holds out his hands and wheels my bike into his shop. He removes the back wheel and sets it on a device that holds it in place while he spins and adjusts the spokes. Rupert stays while I walk to the now open bakery for some sweet buns.

When I return, Rupert and the bike mechanic are standing side by side pointing from my wheel to my tire, wheel to tire. "The problem is…," but his English is not quite up for the job, so he signs with points and shrugs, gesturing at the mechanics of the wheel to signal the problem. The tire bulges and pushes against the wheel causing the wheel to warp. We consider changing the front and back tires and putting a little less air in them, to reduce the pressure. The man shakes his head and frowns. With all the weight I am carrying, it will make little difference and just promote a flat.

"How much," I ask in Thai, but he shakes his head again.

We put my bags back on. My panniers are large, green and beautiful but not designed to slip easily on and off a bike rack. Rupert's are new and well-designed. All he has to do is hold the handle at the back of the pannier—there are two—pull up and pop the top part onto the back rack so it hangs off. He doesn't have to get down on his knees and reach between stiff-backed pannier and dirt and grease-covered bike. He can lift his heavy panniers on and off with one hand, whereas I need six hands to hook and tighten the Velcro straps to the bottom of the rack at the back of the panniers. Having taken them on and off so often these last few days, I am impatient, my fingers weary. Not only that, once I get one pannier on, the bike is lop-sided and the front wheel swings back and forth and nearly knocks me over. *When I get home*, I think, *I'll buy some fancy new ones like Rupert's.*

Where were we? The road widened and spread, an elephant's trunk that unfurled toward Bangkok, while we took two more nights, rode one hundred more kilometres and marveled at the shift from road side fruit stands to Pizza Hut and Kentucky Fried Chicken. In Nakhon Sawan we stayed in a multi-storied, luxury hotel with a hot shower. We ate pizza. It's all okay, we told ourselves, forty-two days in. The edges of where we began or ended and where the lives of the people around us began blurred. I was no longer sure, no longer imagined one time or place or memory over another. There was no struggle for us other than fast traffic and carbon dioxide. We had come a long way, come thousands of miles. Road-weary, we knew what our bikes needed. We would cross the threshold of that other doorway and enter Bangkok, a city that unsettled the nerves, opened us to all that was familiar, commercialized and westernized, yet married to its traditions.

Bikes, Bangkok, Bliss, Thailand, October 21

We walk along the main street, down a few lanes, around a loop, turn left, turn right and wait for the bus. OK. After piling on the bus with hundreds of young Thais, all going to the same place, we hold on or sit for the epic bus ride. Did we eat dinner or are we too excited? I am excited. I am outside myself, outside of everything. Too long have we relied on the day to day and too long have I been inside my head.

The bus jolts to a stop and everyone scrambles off. We glance shyly around at the other round-eyed foreigners onboard, ex-pats who live here. Do we look like them, people out on the town, or do we look alien—our strange tan lines where helmet straps have marked us?

Forget everything I tell myself. Here is freedom without the struggle to find it or feel it.

Everything I need is in my backpack: snacks and insulin. Sometimes I carry it and sometimes Rupert does. As we enter the coliseum, I pass it to him. His shoulders too high for anyone to reach in and grab. Too high to cut off the straps.

This is not like a concert hall at home. Here, we all stream into a space with an open dance floor. In I go, joyous and ready to dance and sing along with a woman just a few years younger than I, but who can sing. I am set free, like a fleet of paper lanterns flying up into the night sky. Do I have a country? I do. I can hear the language of my country in her voice.

That I would be good even if I did nothing...

I want to be good. That is, I want to meet the expectations of the adventurer, of the traveller, not the tourist. Meet my own expectations of myself. Alanis Morissette's inner perfectionist is speaking to mine. Her voice saying that if it all goes wrong, you'll still be ok and good and loved. Whatever failures are in your future, you'll bounce back.

That I would be loved even when I'm not myself
That I would be good even when I'm overwhelmed
That I would be loved even when I am fuming
That I would be loved even when I am clingy

After the concert we take a tuk-tuk back to the guest house rather than endure the bus again. On this trip, there has been nothing like this concert, nothing that so connected me to who I think I am, my feminine angry self.

"Do I stress you out?" she asks. I stress myself out.

…and the held notes of the word clingy and the flute both delicate as breath and strong, fierce, unfaltering. I wanted the music in my head to carry me on. Though Morissette often speaks of love and the other, I often hear her lyrics as a conversation with the self, in my head, keeping me going. Keep going despite my health, the long road, the history of war and colonialism, the dying animals, the natural world in peril, my eternally white and freckled skin, by which I mean, the manifestation of colonialism in the colour of my hair, eyes and skin. What are the deep resources within that I am calling on? What keeps me going? I do not know, but something in Morissette's music speaks to something in me. Her voice, her rage, her honesty, the music itself and how she talks, often to herself.

Bangkok, Thailand, October 22

We stay at the Sawatdee Guest House, in Guest House Quarters, where our neighbours include the Tavee Guesthouse, Backpacker's Lodge, Shanty Lodge, and Original Paradise Guest House. Over the next three days in Bangkok we hop from one to the next, trying each of their different breakfasts, then heading out to absorb all we can of the markets, restaurants, internet cafes, grand palace, hospital, and massage parlours. For those three days, while our bikes are being restored, we not only see Alanis Morissette, but are driven around by an obstinate tuk-tuk driver who wants to take us to places we don't want to go. He stops outside a fancy restaurant while we argue with him. Then he tries to get us out of the tuk-tuk saying "No pay, go," but Rupert refuses. He drives us closer to our guest house but by this time it is after eight so we dine in a strange, Philippine-owned restaurant. Strange because though the staff insists we come in, we feel we've interrupted a private function. The food is basic fried rice, bland for Bangkok where we expect some kind of dietary thrill with every meal.

We visit the famous Emerald Buddha in the palace. It is small, the size of a basketball, but made from one piece of stone. In Laos we learned that the Thais had stolen the statue from Laos. In Bangkok we learn that in fact it originally belonged to the Thais and that the king of Laos was meant to be the king of Thailand upon marrying into Thai royalty. When he returned to Laos to live he took the Buddha with him. The Emerald Buddha, for us, is a history lesson, specifically its veracity or lack of. The Thais now keep the statue safely in the palace temple, out of reach of the Laotians.

We visit one of the green leaf vegetarian restaurants to explore the amazing vegan food, which is basically the same as the food in these restaurants elsewhere, but twice the price. On our way to the Thieves Market a tuk-tuk driver talks us into visiting two Wats and a batik factory. It is a special Buddhist holiday, he says. We have seen more impressive temples along the road and observe no festivities but pay the guy 20 baht. The Batik is beautiful; we buy nothing. Back at the Thieves Market, we buy cloth face masks for our ride out of Bangkok. We also visit a hospital where Rupert is checked out for both stomach woes and the fungus growing on his feet. We buy special cream at the pharmacy. We visit the river side, another market.

Bangkok is a city of chaos, of yellow flowers, bright smiles and capitalism. We love every minute of it. We enjoy chatting with other tourists and visiting the sights and also have fun chatting with locals and talking about their country. On our last day, we visit Thai masseuses.

Rupert is slapped and pulled and pushed on his platform beside me in a busy open-air tent. He chooses the hot wax massage so stinks of tiger balm. The masseuse knees, pokes and elbows me. She pulls, pushes and shakes me loose. We emerge barely able to walk and stumble back to our guest house for cold beers. Maps spread before us, we plan the next leg of the journey south.

Always we were discussing the next part and the next part. In three days. Three days was how long it would take to turn the machines we'd been riding back into bicycles. Bicycle is a French-coined word meaning "two wheels in tandem." Ours were no longer in tandem, nor could our back wheels be called wheels, more ovals, non-circular globes we blumped along on. We needed the high-end bike shop.

"After your first day of cycling, one dream is inevitable. A memory of motion lingers in the muscles of your legs, and round and round they seem to go. You ride through Dreamland on wonderful dream bicycles that change and grow" from The Wheels of Chance, H.G. Wells

Bangkok, Thailand, October 23

We get off the bus outside the Grand Hyatt Erawan Hotel, and walk down the new highway on a wide sidewalk passing the Israeli Embassy, the New Zealand Embassy and the U.S. Embassy, then turn off the main street and follow a smaller road. On the side street, buildings are white-washed but more dilapidated looking with fewer statues, glass and marble carvings. The bike store, tucked along this smaller street, might have been pulled out of Vancouver and dropped in Bangkok to serve our needs. Mountain bikes and racing bikes line the back entrance, while bikes in for repair sit under a tin awning outside. When we see our bikes, we barely recognize them. Not only has someone fixed them—mine with two new tires, straightened wheels, tightened spokes, and Rupert's with a new rear axle, his wheels trued—their immaculate bodies glisten. The red dirt, sand and mud picked up on every unpaved road or shoulder from Vietnam to here is gone. Sure, we've been cleaning them every week or so, checking nuts and bolts for tightness, but this is thorough and detailed. My bike shines turquoise; Rupert's gleams black-speckled white. We circle the bikes a few times, as if they are turquoise and opal gems, then pull ourselves together and enter the busy shop. The shop is cluttered with young guys in racing gear and cycling cleats, and a family of blonde people getting bikes for their two kids. We wait in line, saying, "We're picking up our bikes," while bowing and thanking everyone who passes us. The guy behind the counter is mildly impressed we've come so far on them. He feels certain the new parts will last. We buy some spare spokes and using electric tape, attach them to Rupert's top tube. We pay for the repairs and new tires and after more bowing and thanking (I want to hug everyone, but restrain myself) we head toward the chaos of byways and highways to get back to our guesthouse.

Well into our seventh week of a twelve week trip, in the last three days we have almost spent more money than in all the days before. We'd bought 1300 bhat worth of books, 1200 bhat worth of tickets, spent 850 bhat on medicine and 850 bhat on bike repairs. That didn't include the lodgings for 200 bhat a night, food at about 600 bhat a day. That comes to 66, 000 bhat and doesn't include the price of entering museums, palaces, Wats, or the cost of mad tuk-tuk drivers. Our expenses were supposed to cover up to a maximum of fifteen dollars a day each. In the last three days we'd spent 230 CAD, or eight days living expenses.

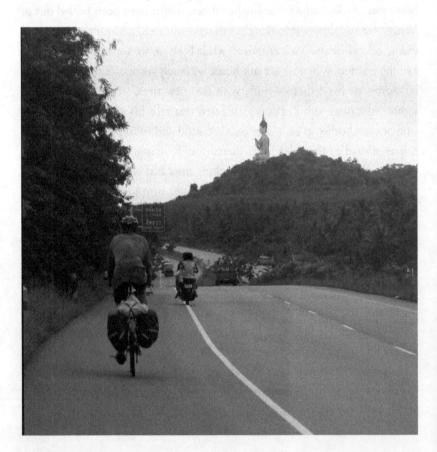

Leaving Bangkok, Thailand, October 24

Our minds on money and time, we cycle out of Bangkok due west toward a floating market off the busy highway. At least, that's the plan. On this smog-filled morning, quiet roads are a kind of dream. Have we ever ridden a quiet road, I wonder, my glasses fogging up because of the cloth face-mask covering my nose and mouth. My ears are clouded with noise, my eyes and skin itch with all the dust and debris thrown at us from trucks and buses, cars, mopeds and the road. The continuous honking-revving-coughing-smoking-stinking chug of traffic wears on us. We pedal on, still in the throes of the city.

Rupert pulls over and I stop behind him. We study our Thai atlas and look at the *Lonely Planet* again. Both indicate that the market is close to Nakhon Pathon. We carry on.

We stop. My skin feels gritty with exhaust. My face, wherever the mask doesn't cover, is gritty too. We buy water and set off again.

We stop in front of a pizza restaurant. It's just past eleven, but we decide to go inside. It looks modern, air conditioned and peaceful. We sit our weary bodies in a booth, a booth of all things, and order lemon juice and pizzas. We chat with an American couple and their two boys at a neighbouring table.

"We wanted to bring the kids so they could see this country," the woman says. "We both travelled here when we were your age."

The couple is only in their mid-thirties, a little older than we are, but they seem much older. They seem cool and grown up and capable of taking care of kids. They are heading to the market as well, but are going further south to Samut Songkhram, apparently the shorter way. They travel by car.

I check the atlas "You're right," I say. "If we'd headed more southwest we could have gotten off this awful road sooner and would have been closer to the market." I shrug. It is too late. We'd have to back-track too far. From where we are, the only road available goes directly to Nakhon Pathon. We are only about thirty kilometres from it, though it seems like we are still in the thick of Bangkok.

As we leave the sanctity of the café to get back on the road, I wave to the family. I feel a longing, a magical connection to them. A couple and two kids. The kids are seven and nine, and excited about being in Thailand. Rupert and I are twenty-eight. I could be a mom instead of a dirty woman on a bike. Rupert could be a dad. The couple seem so established, somehow. Do they represent something I am missing or might miss? Something we might be heading toward? They look as if they have real jobs and real lives. I feel like I've met an older sister out here, in the wilds of Asia.

How do these small moments, these fragments of memory, grab onto me like this? How is it possible that a half an hour in a cool restaurant can stay with me? I didn't know where we were going on that specific day and I didn't know where we were going at the end of the trip. We were on the cusp, in the space of the adventures and the future. The couple and their boys seemed to represent one or many of those possibilities. The notion that we would go home, get jobs and build our lives and that might include buying a house or car, getting a dog, having a kid. I was caught between where I was and where I might be going.

We finally get a break. The city disappears and the road opens to trees. It lasts less than ten kilometers and we are back in traffic as we approach

Nakhon Pathon. Though we are further from the market, something about this town appeals. We find a hotel behind the bus depot, where we go to check on buses to the floating market. One leaves at six the next morning. The hotel is seven stories high, not much to look at, but we don't care. I just want to lug my bags up, go back for my bike, lug my bike, drop everything and collapse. My FoMo (Rupert's name for my condition—fear of missing out) has me in the shower before I manage to fall asleep and ready to go wandering before darkness sets in.

Nakhon Pathom, believed to be the oldest city in Thailand, was conquered by Angkor in the early eleventh-century. In what looks to be the centre of town, sits the 127 metre orange-tiled Phra Pathom Chedi, the tallest Buddhist monument in the world. In November there will be a fair in celebration of the Chedi but tonight, it seems, preparations for a party are underway. We walk through a huge night-market to get to the Chedi and attached museum. On the way through the market, I spot a health food store.

"I know I'm obsessed with food but how long has it been since I've been in a health food store?" I ask Rupert, dragging him in so he will okay some frivolous purchases—yummy looking cookies and unsweetened yogurt, some kind of tofu jerky stuff.

"Sebun, erebun, ii kibu-un," slips out of my mouth. The theme song for 7-11 in Japan rings through me as we continue our walk around the town. I am searching, seeking something in the way of food comfort, or a new piece of clothing, I am hankering for a change in what I put in my mouth or on my body. I want some kind of sensory satisfaction. Want to be sated in a way that I can't pinpoint. This is the aftereffect of Bangkok.

"Sebun, erebun, ii kibu-un" I sing when I see the familiar convenience store. "Seven, Eleven, good feeling."

"There just something about popcorn," I say to Rupert as we enter but he is more interested in a Big Gulp than stale yellow corn.

We learned in Japan that though 7-11 has made it to Asia, the food inside has not. No Big Gulps, no jumbo bags of chips and no Twizzler sticks. That's okay. We don't really want those. In Thailand there are no rice balls with seaweed or salmon either, of course, though that would be amazing. I'd love some 7-11 *onigiri*. Each of these chain stores follows its own country's tastes. Apparently, Thai youths have a thing for popcorn. Also, I find pastries that look something like samosas but discover, on my first bite, that indeed they are potato-based, but sweetened with honey. To Rupert's delight, the 7-11 in Nakhon Pathon sells corn dogs.

"Why is it," I ask as we head toward a funky looking boutique at the back of our hotel, "that we are now craving home food? Has Bangkok ruined us for the rest of the trip?" I also want to look at clothing in cute shops. Perhaps our nearness to the beach is making me crazy.

"Food is a big thing," Rupert says. "We craved western food in Japan. You are just sick of sweet snacks and fried rice."

On our way back to the hotel, I pop into the 7-11 again. We need a couple of big bottles of water and I discover, to my delight, that they have diet coke. I buy two cans. One to drink right away and one for later, when I am really desperate. "Funny," I say, "Diet Coke has no nutritional value or calories, and I've bought two for when I'm desperate."

"You're crazy." Rupert simply says, pulling me homeward. No more shopping, no more silly chit chat. He is road-weary and bed-ready. It's only nine so I'll have to stay up and entertain myself until post-injection. Maybe I'll play solitaire with our ratty deck of cards and sip a Diet Coke. "There wasn't even Diet Coke in Japan." I say. Rupert grunts in reply.

Reading Kim Thúy's Ru *while camping on French Beach, Vancouver Island. Thinking about the refugee, the immigrant. My desire to have few possessions. In my twenties I began buying laptop computers because when I moved from Nanaimo to Vancouver my computer took up my entire car. How could I escape*

with my valuables if the computer fills all the space? Now married with a kid and dog what would I take if I had to escape? Son, dog, books, computer. I have a memory of leaving Rhodesia by boat, of dark faces in the night, of holding something in my lap. But what did I hold? A blanket or toy? My sister's hand? We were not refugees. We were leaving because my parents no longer felt safe. Because they could not befriend the Africans without being judged for it. A list of the dead my dad found years later in a history book. Were they names of people he knew? What people? Is this a memory or a story I've made up with an image tied to it? Left because two young daughters and no sense of a future.

Lom Kao, Thailand, October 14

I lie down to sleep while Rupert goes to find a doctor. The conjunctivitis I woke with this morning needs more than eye drops. Rupert has it too, but mine is worse. Maybe the girl at the irrigation pool had been trying, too late, to warn us not to swim in the water buffalo-pee-infested pool.

Rupert returns and reports on his visit. The doctor has given us penicillin and eye drops. He also laughed at our Doxycycline, the drug we take to fend off malaria, saying Thais overuse it. We decide to keep taking it, since we have plenty of bites but no sign, thus far, of malaria. I crash for the rest of the day, my eyes oozing onto the pillow and my muscles weary.

In the evening we walk up the dead-dark street from our guest house into the hustle and bustle of evening market life and right on the corner, across from the video store and next to the ice cream parlour sits a vegan restaurant. We take plates and scoop spoonfuls of food, all of it meat-shaped but made from wheat gluten and god knows what other meat substitutes. I select a "drumstick" coated in thick red paste, some sticky rice and some other meat also coated in the same paste. Rupert picks a potato looking thing and some green curry and we sit at a low plastic table. The oldest matron of the establishment yells at a child of ten who quickly drops two cups of water on our plastic table, then follows moments later with a pitcher. We can see the bottled water in the corner from which she's filled our cups and jug so it is safe to drink. Our guts have acclimatized to Asia now; stomach problems have hardly been a concern for weeks. We drink enough water and sweat during the day to flush out any "friends" we make along the way.

I bite into my "drumstick" excited about this vegetarian protein. I'm so happy to not have to ask and ensure and double check and have Rupert taste test that I forget for the moment about my eyes. I quickly discover the red paste is pure, tongue-searing, spice. Red hot peppers with a little cayenne added for flavour. I love the taste and share with Rupert but my mouth and lips burn. The other patrons and servers at the counter are all quiet. I take a second bite, thinking it is best to eat quickly so I can finish before the fire engulfs me. While biting, I notice all eyes glued to us, watching our faces flame red. Thank goodness our server anticipated our agony and provided us with lots of water. My red hot drumstick is nothing compared to Rupert's green curry.

In Thailand we are easy with each other and ourselves. Despite my sore eyes. Our hard edges, softened. It is more familiar, more westernized.

And my blood sugars? Have I spoken about highs? The thirst and crankiness. The danger of riding with high sugars because my body would burn fat for energy and risk ketoacidosis.

Rest Day, Thailand, October 15

I recall three whole days in Vientiane while Rupert slept and recovered from an illness while I entertained myself in museums and cafes. For me, a single night's rest. Why? Goopy eyed, I unglue my eyelids and we are up, packed and out hunting for breakfast before the third crow of the rooster. Is it because of my innate restlessness or because Rupert doesn't allow me to be sick? I have a feeling it's the former. My sugars have leapt up to 10.1, the ideal being between 4.5-6, so sugars in addition to infected eyes are not only playing off each other, but also making my temperament less than ideal.

We ride the mere thirteen kilometres to Lom Sak, the next town over. Technically, this is a rest day so we are just moving for change, not to cover any distance. After a rolling forty-minute bike ride, we arrive and after another hour of circling and circling we find a place to stay on a quiet back street. We stop at the front house which looks like a small rickety club house. The buildings are all single story and the front house, where we check in, get bedding and towels, has three or four, maybe five men in it and a snotty-nosed boy who eyes our every move. Key in hand we move to a numbered room in the courtyard. It looks like a nicely painted prison without the gates and bars. We don't need to shower, so I rest on the bed with a damp handkerchief on my face. I want to just lie there until the throbbing in my eyes and the bleary muckiness fade. Rupert wants to get out and walk around. This is such a total shift from the norm. It's almost lunch time and he doesn't want to go without me so I pull myself from the bed and slip my feet into sandals. We lock our bikes in the room. Without them it starts to feel like a rest day.

I begin to wonder if restlessness is a form of loneliness. I wonder if homesick-ness wasn't catching up to us in our conversation with the Thai kickboxer who could speak Japanese, in our swim and walk with the kids at the temple in the making, in Rupert's long chat with the doctor. Were we searching for belonging? "Everyone longs for a secret door, an opening to a world beyond loneliness—it is part of the human condition" writes Kathleen Winter in Boundless. Though we were together, we were also boundless, and alone. We had longed to fit in in Japan, but gaijin perhaps never do. The intricacies of a deep understanding of all the cultures and languages we met in the three months we travelled were beyond us.

Rupert finds the local vegetarian restaurant, with me following along. This time we go easy on the red-paste coated food. We also quickly make new friends, two girls named Mimi, who is seventeen, and Taang, twenty-six. We promise to come back for dinner. Even if we hadn't befriended the girls, we would go back. Eating in an all vegan restaurant is the closest thing to nirvana I've found thus far in life.

After dinner, Mimi and Taang take us on a tour on their mopeds. We stop at Taang's house to switch mopeds for her father's truck. They want to take us somewhere, we aren't sure where, we just go along.

"We go see famous statue," says Mimi.

The four of us squeeze into the front seat of the truck and Taang throws it into gear and barrels down a dark, dirt road.

"We should have brought a flashlight," Mimi says.

Rupert looks out the window as Taang turns off the "highway" onto an even more treacherous dirt road. At the closed gate at the bottom, she stops the truck and we all pile out.

"This is the entrance," says Taang, walking toward the small hut with a ticket vendor sitting inside. We listen to the murmur of their voices. I note a lot of head shaking. Taang comes back. "It closed at eight."

We pile back into the truck. Mimi and Taang talk a mile a minute and then look at Rupert and me.

"Where we go now?" asks Mimi. The tires on the truck spin out and the rear end sinks deeper into mud.

"Oh," Mimi and Taang say in unison.

Rupert gets out and I follow. We push and push, but the truck is stuck. The ticket vendor comes out of his hut with a muddy plank of wood. He and Rupert wedge it under the back tire while Taang revs the engine. With a loud splat, the wheel pops out and the plank breaks.

"Kaap kun kaa," I say, bowing slightly as we cram ourselves back in and the vendor tosses the plank into the bushes.

After more chattering, we drive back to Taang's, retrieve the mopeds out of the garage and park the truck. Rupert and I drive one, the girls the other.

"We sing karaoke," says Mimi as they speed off and we follow.

The girls lead us into the parking lot of a fancy hotel. Walking up the vast staircase to the entrance, I wonder if we are appropriately dressed in our only "civilian" outfit. My rayon pants feel a bit thin and washed out. I am also wearing a blue t-shirt that has been hand-washed every week for the past five weeks. Rupert wears deathly pale, faded beige khakis and an equally pale, green, button-up shirt. At least we are clean. We sit in a booth in an almost deserted lounge.

"You want drink?" asks Taang, who then goes off to the bar, returning with beers for us and a couple of Cokes for her and Mimi. A song book is under her arm.

Had we just arrived to Southeast Asia the idea of karaoke might have daunted us. But, we are experts. We have been living in Japan. The choices in English are the limited familiar few we've seen in Japan. I sing Celine Dion's *Titanic* theme song and Rupert sings the Police's "Roxanne." There is a plethora of Beetles' song, which we sing along with the girls. We attempt a Thai pop song, but it is too fast and our attempts make everyone giggle. Rupert keeps up the attempt, his expressions of mock-sincerity making the three of us giggle even more.

The girls won't let us pay for a thing, and drop us off at home before midnight.

I remember these young women because they were like so many people we met along the way during those two and a half years in Asia. These fleeting, essential connections. Time with people who are essentially the same as us. Young women I taught or spent a day with but did not really get to know. We were transient. We were picked up and pocketed, then dropped. We picked up and pocketed people too. They shaped and changed our relationship to the other.

As promised, we return to the veggie restaurant for breakfast and lean our loaded bikes against a pole outside where we can keep an eye on them. My eyes are weepy, but I can see and keep them clear for hours at a time. Each time we stop, I will put drops in. Mimi and Taang see our bikes for the first time and they are impressed. Taang leans mine against her body and can't believe its weight. Mimi circles Rupert's, one hand on his seat the height of her shoulders. They then lead us into the restaurant to help us choose our food. This being our fourth spicy, vegan meal in two days, our mouths (and stomachs) are accustomed. We load up our Tupperware with extras for lunch.

After breakfast and just before the difficult goodbyes, Taang disappears on her moped and comes back on a bicycle.

"How many modes of transport does the girl have?" Rupert quietly asks before we all ride to the bus depot, Mimi on Tang's back fender.

We know the day holds mountains, mammoth mountains, so have decided to bus to the top of the worst, about 50 km, and ride from there.

The girls give us gifts—two Chinese back scratchers and a small vial of anti-itch cream for mosquito bites. Mimi kisses us goodbye. We wave to them from the bus, warmed by their friendship and kindness. It feels like we've had a short holiday with old friends, which is just what we needed, a little distraction from the road and the sometimes mundane pattern of pack-cycle-unpack-shower-sleep. We've made friends, the perfect friends for long travellers. Two girls who ask very little of us, but give so much of themselves. We are warmed by their loveliness, softened. They remind us of students in Japan. They also remind us to nurture our own kindness with each other, and others we meet.

Being alone makes me think about how hard aloneness is. I crave it but also shrink within it. It is harder now to separate my alone-time from mother-guilt at leaving my family so I can be alone. I believe we are more vulnerable as individuals. In Japan, in big groups of other ex-pats, the temptation was to forget the larger culture around us. One time a group of us went on a road

trip, but we were respectful, we didn't forget to remember where we were. Is that entirely true? Maybe we did forget, maybe sometimes we stayed inside our language-culture-bubble. That's what getting lost in the group is, you lose awareness of the world outside the group. Which brings up colonialism and the pressures placed on the rebellious individual in a colonial collective. The one person who befriends the outsiders becomes an outsider. Or the one Japanese person travelling with the foreign pack can become an outsider to her Japanese friends.

Danang, Vietnam, September 23

Riding to the Laos consulate, we notice a young man on a bright, shiny, yellow motorbike following us. When we turn into the Laos Visa office parking area, he follows. As we settle our bikes, drink water and dig for papers, he approaches us in his dress shirt and black pants. He smiles and tells us his name is Tuan, then offers to watch our bikes while we fill out papers. We agree. We can see them from inside anyway. After several corrections and short, gestured discussions, we learn that our Visas will take a day. Outside Tuan wants to know our plans. When we tell him we've decided to ride on to Hoi An for the night he is delighted. "But first," he says, "you must come to my house for lunch."

He revs the engine of his yellow motorbike and drives a slow twenty kilometres while we follow down to the main street, toward the bus depot. He stops outside a fan shop. We lock our bikes together under the awning and follow him through the bright shop, packed with varying sized fans, air conditioners and a few cleaning supplies stocked against one wall. Through an opening in a long dark curtain I can see a small living room and dining table. The kitchen consists of a kettle and hotplate.

"Come," Tuan says, and we follow him. His aunt, we guess, and brother or cousin, sit on the couch watching TV. The fan shop is quiet and the dark cool back room or living space welcome, though crowded. Tuan leaves us with his relatives and pops to the store for an array of meatless meats. It is the lunar festival so the Vietnamese are eating only vegetarian food.

Rupert asks a few questions, but we only get nods in response so fall silent. Tuan's aunt smiles at us but she does not speak. When Tuan reappears, his aunt hops up for plates and cutlery.

I am excited but cautious about the food, so when Tuan says, "Here try this, it is not meat, but we call chicken," I look at him warily. His aunt, standing over the table, laughs out loud, shaking her head.

"No. No. Trust me, this is not really meat."

I look sideways at Rupert, his mouth full already. He gives a small nod. This sends Tuan and his aunt into further fits of laughter.

"You more like the monks." Tuan says. "We Vietnamese, we really don't like the Lunar festival because we have to go hungry." He decides I am more pure than the Monks and meat-starved Vietnamese of these incessant Lunar days.

We discuss our plans over tea. Tuan wants to help. His uncle drives a bus so he can get info on the buses for when we return the next day. Since we are heading toward Hoi An, Tuan wants to guide us part of the way and take us to Marble Mountain. We shrug our compliance.

We follow Tuan due east toward China Beach, then turn onto the highway heading south. We pass the industrial part of Danang with motorbike and auto shops. Buses and trucks in pieces line the lane that runs along the highway. Tuan leads, going slowly, or looping around when he gets too far ahead. After about thirteen kilometres he turns off to the right, down a dirt road. At the end of the road, a low hill, and over to the far right, a cluster of buildings that could be small shops. Tuan points up a narrow path, where there are caves. Rupert and I decide we will take turns, so I stand with the bikes while he and Tuan take a look. While they are gone, I visit with a few hens and a rooster and watch a few monks go in and out of the buildings across the way. Rupert returns looking less than impressed and it is my turn. After the second cave Tuan and the guide want us to climb the mountain. This time we shrug our non-compliance and tell him we need to go.

"It is already 2:30 and we want to see some of Hoi An. We'll only have today," Rupert says, hunching a little as if to seem smaller.

Tuan eventually agrees, but wants to hire a photographer to take our pictures. He gets on his bike and rides back to town to hire a professional photographer. We sit and wait with the chickens. A young monk who seems a cross between a Hell's Angel and bald punk teenager sits in the shade of his small hut playing loud music. Occasionally he pops his head out to stare at us.

The photographer arrives and takes pictures of Tuan and me, Rupert and Tuan, Rupert and me and the three of us together. Finally, we leave. Our hope is to ride back tomorrow, pick up our passports, visit Tuan, buy snacks and get on our way to Laos.

"Come to my shop tomorrow," Tuan says as we climb onto our bikes.

We nod in unison and wave. "See you in the afternoon," we shout back. "Thanks."

Sometimes I imagine for a moment that Tuan will read this. That would be amazing. That fills me with terror as well. How one-sided this is. How my assumptions, how my writing, suggests things that in the living aren't there. He looked young and sweet. We did too. The sun shone. The world full of expecta-tion. Morissette sings "Enough about me, let's talk about you for a while. Enough about you, let's talk about life for a while."

As of 1999 Hoi An was a UNESCO World Heritage Site and a well pre-
served ancient trading port. We cycle into the town late in the afternoon and
after coasting through a small suburban landscape enter an active cultural
museum with French colonial hotels and shops on narrow streets. Paper
lanterns hang from shop front to shop front and quiet little restaurants and
pubs are tucked down ever narrower lanes and alleys. We check into the
first hotel we see and after clambering up three stories and dumping our
bags on the stone-tiled floor, crawl through the large windows to stand on
our narrow balcony and take in the town. Picture New Orleans. Picture
immaculate, white washed fronts and gray, decaying backs. Picture old
Western towns where the buildings are ornate at the front but unadorned
and plain at the back.

"Between the seventh and tenth centuries Hoi An, under the name
Lam Ap Pho, was the centre of the spice trade," I read to Rupert as he
relaxes on the bed for a minute. "Between the sixteenth and seventeenth-
centuries Chinese, Japanese, Dutch and Indian traders were using the Thu
Bon River for trade."

He sighs.

From our balcony we can see hordes of people down below. The autumn
lunar festival has packed Hoi An with visitors. This represents the highest
concentration of white faces we have seen since a farewell party in Japan
back in June. We don't have much time before dark, so I put on sandals
and pull Rupert out to join the throngs.

"Hoi An is famous for the colonial architecture as well as Chinese and
Japanese buildings," I say in my tour-guide voice. "A melding of Vietnamese, Chinese and Japanese architecture," I add, with a head wiggle.

Rupert sighs but follows. It is late in the day so time and light are precious. Hoi An is also known for its plethora of clothing shops but we've already decided to bypass them.

Down on the street, a parade has begun. Two children push a handcart carrying a drum, pushing and drumming while three others dance in a Chinese dragon costume. They dance into a store and a child wearing a mask that looks like a happy Buddha collects money from the shop owner. The festival is to bring good luck to business owners. As the children move on to the next street, the pedestrians begin to move again. As if reanimated, they enter shops gathering abandoned conversations on their way.

I pull out of the throng to lean against a post card shop wall when a woman approaches. "You need film?"

My camera whirrs, rewinding the finished roll. I nod.

She leads Rupert and me down the next street to a film shop and on to her own clothing shop. Beautifully made shirts and blouses, skirts and dresses hang above me, draped partly over Rupert's head. The colours and fabrics are gorgeous. When did I last look in a mirror? I wear lip balm, the extent of my makeup. How can I even hope to reject this hard-sell approach? Shirt after shirt, dress after dress is draped on me. Rupert keeps saying "No, I don't need it," thinking of the bikes and their already heavy loads, but it gets him nowhere with the flock of young women pushing this and that shirt and material up against him. "Oh, this one good with your blue eyes," one woman says. We leave after ordering two shirts for me and a pair of pants and a shirt for Rupert. One of the shirts will be a Christmas gift for my sister.

"Pretty good restraint," I say to Rupert, taking his hand and squeezing it as we finally walk out.

He laughs and squeezes back, relieved to get out of the store but, I think, secretly happy about the shirts. All our new clothes will be ready for us, made by hand, by morning.

Back on the street, we bump into Ann, the English woman we met in Dong Hoi about five days earlier. She is surprised to see us. "Hoy, I thought you'd be in Laos by now!"

"Ann! Oh, we got sidetracked with Visas in Danang so decided to come here for the night."

We find a restaurant to have a drink. Just as we settle at a table and order beer the entire city goes dark. All the lanterns and sound systems running at once for all the small festivities around town strain have strained the generators. When they stop, the streets go instantly quiet, as people hesitantly make their way, whispering and tiptoeing. We sit by candlelight and catch up with Ann and her adventures while sharing ours, immersed in a small halo of light.

Later, the generators fail again so we walk in the pitch dark to the famous Japanese bridge. Despite the lack of light, we can see the ornate sculpture of the outside walls and roof. Made for pedestrians as a way to link the Japanese and Chinese sides of Hoi An in the 1700s, the bridge is a narrow temple over the churning river. An homage to Japanese and Chinese architecture, to the long connection between these two powerful cultures. From the Chinese or Vietnamese end, we step into the enclosed bridge, into utter darkness above a narrow river. The usual decay on the entranceway shows in faded and crumbling walls but it seems that the entrance is cement and patched on more recently to bolster the existing stone. The decorations on the roof are similar to those on the many temples and pagodas we've visited in Japan but this bridge is said to be the only known Japanese bridge with a Buddhist Pagoda at one end. It reminds me of the close ties, historically, between Japan and Vietnam. Only forty years after it was built, the Tokugawa Shogunate called all Japanese back to Japan and closed their borders. That the bridge remains, impresses me even more. Though we walk to the centre and look out to the churned up muddy water below, we don't cross over to the other side where it is utterly dark.

Back in the throes of the festivities, we note the low buildings and narrow cobbled pedestrian-wide paths. Few mopeds go by as the streets are packed with children and visitors. The children continue their parade for hours with floats depicting Buddha, warriors and goddesses going up and down the busy streets. Drums pound wildly and people cheer. We walk with a parade of children wearing white shirts, black pants and red or yellow paper hats. They carry paper and tinfoil circles with the Vietnamese flag's star in the centre. The street opens up to the wide town square where a stage is set for a dragon dance competition. The backdrop to the stage is a giant picture of Uncle Ho holding a child in his arms. The city parties on long after we return to our room and fall to bed for short spasms of sleep interrupted by partiers, or power cuts, which change our fan-cooled haven to a roasting oven.

Hoi An was a brief pause. We were readying to leave Vietnam. We immersed ourselves in colour; in children and roosters; in sun setting over the low town and lanterns hanging from store front to store front; in Colonial French architecture, and Chinese, Japanese, Vietnamese. The world a cracked oyster shell. There cannot always be such piercing doubt. Sometimes we must just shop or laugh or drink a beer. This is still, and only, the beginning. There are miles of villages and road, river and ocean, sand and sunset, flat tires and aching limbs to go. Travellers and tourists, we are a long way from the long road of home. Can you unpack all of the learning from one time to use in another?

Danang, Vietnam, September 24

"Dnang me, Dnang me, they ought to get a rope and hang me "
   —by Roger Miller quoted in the movie *Good Morning Vietnam*

We collect our passports and ride into the thick of Danang to find a book store, a bank and a post office. I want to mail the new clothing home. We ride along the river, heading into the Chinese part of Danang where food stalls abound, bakeries, and magazine stalls, none with English titles. On the corner of one street I find a tour office. We pop in to get bus information. We know Tuan is looking into this but decide to check for ourselves. The disappointing news is that buses to Savannakhet are 30 USD and don't go until Sunday at eight p.m. Sunday? Now I understand that little ditty Robin Williams sings in *Good Morning Vietnam*. Ready to leave, we are trapped for three more days.

"There must be a bus," I say.

"She seemed pretty clear," Rupert says.

"Should we ride back to Hue and bus from there?"

"Could do but remember the huge mountain passes the bus lumbered over getting here?"

We decide to have a beer, then go and meet Tuan.

A groggy Tuan, sporting an impressive bed head, greets us. It is afternoon, I think, shouldn't he be in school? He quickly gets on the phone to find out about buses—120,000 dong—but none leave until Sunday night, confirming what we already know.

"Maybe we should bus back to Dong Hoi, then change for Lao Bao," I offer.

Tuan doesn't think there will be buses from Dong Hoi.

While Rupert and I sit and try to figure out what to do, Tuan takes off to buy lunch. He shakes his head at our offered money. When he gets back, Rupert puts some money on the table and sticks the hot sauce on top of it. The vegetarian restrictions still stand. This couldn't be a better time for us to be hanging out with locals, I decide, as Tuan opens the bags of assorted meatless meats and gets plates.

Once lunch is out of the way, Tuan says he'll find us a hotel.

"Don't worry," Rupert says, thinking we can ride around on our bikes until we find one.

"No. I find you good place. I quote you real price."

"Of course," I say, surprised by his dark look. "We just..."

"We're just happy looking at a few places and finding one we like," Rupert says.

"No. I will find you one. It is good." Tuan turns his back to us as he dials a number on the phone. I glance at Rupert and shrug.

"I quote you real price," he says, looking back at us before trying another number.

A sense of unease settles over me, but over what, I'm not sure. We are independent, want to control our movement and decisions. Rupert and I sit in silence as Tuan quietly talks on the phone. I don't know what to do. Should we help clean up lunch, should we walk into the store and look around? I feel a growing lump in my throat, a desire to break out. Eventually, he finds one, directly across the street. His face is still dark as we all walk to the hotel together. Tuan escorts us to check out a room and decides it is fine. We agree to see him in a few hours for a visit to the beach.

We just want to get out of Vietnam. Something of the chained monkey coming over me. Years from now, and for years, I will best remember Vietnam. It will stand out in memories and dreams, in poems. It has a cultural link to North

America, to the college teacher who was a draft dodger during the Vietnam War. Movies, music, the influx of post-war Vietnamese, and friends, poetry. The hippy movement in North America, the romance of it all. Janis Joplin, Simon and Garfunkle, songs written and sung as a result of the war. It was the struggle, too, the sharp curve of learning. The country's determination to be itself despite colonialism and war. I even seemed to have some regard for Uncle Ho, as he was called, because…why? Socialism, I guess. The ability to reduce crime or AIDs through some form of love/dominance. The many movies in the 1980s on the Vietnam war so that place names were familiar. Characters, known. But stuck in Danang the sun rises and sets, our heads bowed down, bobbed up in waiting. Wanting it to be different.

Rupert and I leave our money belts in the hotel and walk over to the fan shop with towels and snacks, but plans have changed. The day has turned overcast and Tuan decides it is too cold for the beach. We will go on a river boat dinner cruise instead.

The boat is large and red with two dragon heads at the front. A quiet evening, the boat sits at dock waiting for potential guests. The view from on board is of a mud-brown, slow-moving river. Though it is cloudy, or because it is, the sunset turns the entire sky pink, then blue-orange. Long, Tuan's university friend, joins us and we relax into conversation about school. They both study computer science. The waiter drops menus on our table after taking a long look at Rupert. We glance at the menus and Rupert, ignoring the waiter, decides we need more money. This is no cheap boat. He and Tuan leave for our hotel while Long and I talk, on and off, about the weather and our trip so far. We are both more at ease with the other two around.

Rupert and Tuan return just before the boat leaves dock. We stand outside to watch the city slip away. Danang is not a beautiful city. The river, buildings and streets all appear mud-coloured. The boat, in contrast, is almost gaudy in its red paint and gold trim. In our beachwear, shorts and t-shirts, Rupert and I feel as gaudy as the boat. We are certainly not dressed for a luxury dinner cruise. Forced to stay three more days in Vietnam, we are as muddled as the mud, trapped on a treadmill, running in place.

For dinner, Rupert and I share one dish between us. The prices are higher than anything we've seen so far. Not expensive by Canadian standards but way beyond our budget or the cash we have on hand.

"This boat is pretty expensive." Rupert says, dropping hints. "We'll just have water, and stir fried vegetables and rice."

The waiter is full of attitude but can't convince us to order drinks. He has more success with Long and Tuan who order three dishes and a beer each.

The boat chugs along for an hour or so. Just before it ties up, the waiter brings the bill. He hands it to Rupert who picks it up, casually calculates what we owe and puts our share on the table. He then hands the bill to Tuan and Long, setting it on the table between them.

Their bill is over 240, 000 dong. Ours cost $13.35 and theirs adds up to double.

Long, Tuan and the waiter get into a long discussion. I suspect the waiter egged them on all evening to order expensive dishes since the foreigners would pay for them. The bill sitting in front of them is a shock. After a few more minutes, money exchanges hands. I can't see what they pay, but it is less than what Rupert paid. The waiter glares at us and walks off.

I make eye-contact with both guys and smile, "That was lovely," I say, hoping to encourage conversation or a comment. But I fail.

Our plans for the evening are ruined.

"We have no money," Tuan says.

I cringe, wishing, somehow, we'd had the foreknowledge to have exchanged more of our money or at least been open, all of us, from the get-go. It is obvious that we have an advantage over them, but what we don't have is much disposable cash. This is a tiresome conundrum and it puts a rift between us that cannot be mended.

Once docked, we decide to go for a tour of the city with Rupert and me on one moped, the guys on the other. We follow them, but every few minutes they pull over to stare at us and sulk. Tuan is so miserable he barely speaks. My impatience with him grows each time we stop to chat about where to go next and we are met with silence and his long sad pale face. We pull over again.

"Well, where now?" Rupert asks.

Tuan just shakes his head. He's out of ideas. The weather is not great, and we are all out of money so going for a drink is also out of the question. Long just shrugs.

"Well," I sigh, "let's just say goodnight." I am done, done, and ready to walk away. I begin to swing my leg off the bike, but Tuan pipes up, his voice edgy, on the verge of anger.

"No. We will take you to hotel."

We've seen Tuan's dark side, and I feel a rising tide of shame and frustration wash over me as well. We aren't exactly the dream tourists, I gather. We aren't the boon Tuan needs. However, since the next day, September 25, is Rupert's birthday, we will meet them for drinks in the evening.

When I think about the costs in terms of dollars, and in terms of what we spend on a meal now, it feels pathetic. In a small zip-lock-like Japanese folder I have a few tiny mementos gathered along the way. My blood sugar log book. Photos of a tranquil bathroom in Thailand. Postcards. A small brown notebook from Japan, into which I've stapled pages from a small calendar for the months we were away on the front page. A list of what was in our panniers

that I made when packing and pairing down. On the front cover, the name of two bike repair shops in Bangkok that I found on the slow internet in small town Thailand. Poem fragments. A list of all our expenses for the first few days, so we could track and get a sense of how far the money would go. It was September 24. We had Japanese Yen in traveller's cheques and bills and we had a credit card. The credit card would not once work. 120,000 dong was the cost of a night's accommodation. We spent that on food alone. There were no bank machines. But this feels, years later, like excuses. The fact is we didn't have the money on us. With us, on the boat. Quiet fact.

Danang, Vietnam, September 25

I WANT IT THAT WAY. TELL ME WHY? AIN'T NOTHIN' BUT A HEART ACHE,
TELL ME WHY?

"What the hell?" Rupert bolts up. Music blares up and down the halls
of our guest house. We are the only guests. After putting on his shorts
and sticking his head out the door, he discovers the two young girls, who
checked us in the day before, dancing in the entrance way to the Backstreet
Boys. He comes back in and slams the door.

"Oh my," I say, getting up. I wander down the hall looking for the stereo.
It is in the closet off the dining room. I walk in and turn the music off.

"It's five in the morning," Rupert says when I return.

TELL ME WHY. AIN'T NOTHING BUT A HEART ACHE. TELL ME WHY?

I sit up and check the time. Six. I hop into the shower. By the time I get
out I've decided we are moving hotels. We don't feel comfortable being so
close to Tuan. We realize suddenly how awkward things have been, how
hard we've been trying. We feel like our movement is restricted by his
scowling eyes. We feel trapped enough being stuck in Danang and Vietnam when we are ready to be on the road. We are wound up and need to
gain some control. Blaring music at five a.m. is the last straw. We get our
money back, pack our things and move to a hotel of our own choosing.
The atmosphere of the night before has put us off. I feel badly for the guys
and their lack of money but they pulled us onto that fancy boat which
none of us could afford. After the boat ride, anything we said violently

offended or angered Tuan. He'd glare at us in pale silence, refusing to respond even to simple suggestions or questions like "Let's go to the beach," or "How far to a park?" We missed the nuance, clearly, of what was expected of us. Moving meant he'd be angrier, I was sure, but it also meant we'd be a little more in control.

Our new hotel is, in the end, a dollar more a night, but we have a big comfortable bed and the owner will let us check out late before heading out on the bus at no extra charge.

"Let's go to the beach," I say to Rupert as he stands in the middle of our new room looking miserable and sweating after carrying his stuff up. We get towels, swimsuits, books and snacks and hop on our bikes to pedal to China Beach. We know it is jellyfish season, but we don't care.

On the way out, near the intersection we took to get to Hoi An, I spot a bakery. "Let's get a cake!" Rupert seems a bit glum and down in the dumps for a birthday boy.

The mud-coloured streets of yesterday glisten brightly as we head off the main street toward the beach. More mud than sand, China Beach is not beautiful. During the war GIs came here for R&R, but since the war it has become, or reverted to, a fishing village, the beach littered with glass, plastic and old lures. We push our bikes down the sand to a clean patch of beach with a tree for shade and settle in for the morning. Trapped here, waiting for the bus, we have limited options but we probably need to simply relax.

I try to control my restlessness since, having decided how we will get to Laos, we have to stick with our decision. Tuan's negative energy hangs over us and exacerbates our weariness of the country. It also heightens our own sense of guilt. We are on the beach, he is broke: the irony of it all is not lost on either of us.

"Are you surprised by how little that meal cost, now all these years later," I ask Rupert.

He is home sick from work. We've had lunch. I'm stuck. Disturbed by the memory of this encounter.

"But there were so many facets to what was going on," he says.

I locate him in our own story: After having met the young girl. After we started to rest on the peak of bridges so we could see people approach. After Yung in Hue.

"Where was it that security guard at a bus depot approached us and yelled out twenty dollars?"

"Hue," I say, "I remember, we just rode away."

"For me it was the climax, the exemplar of how we equalled money. Everyone at that bus depot saw us, each shouted out a larger and larger number—20, 30 dollars, then Where you going."

"Yeah and the posted price to Danang was less than a dollar."

"It wore us down. And Tuan was not straight forward. Remember his friend saying he didn't really understand him. We couldn't shake ourselves loose."

"But it was hardly any money. I'm stuck."

"Remember you got that tax bill in Japan? We tracked every dollar we spent. Were there bank machines?"

"No. All we had were Japanese yen traveller's cheques. We'd put some money on our visa for emergencies but it never worked."

"That's right. Yeah. It is easy to think we were being cheap because, if we'd paid for theirs, a forty dollar dinner is nothing now."

"But that was four days' budget," I add. "Forty dollars now with us both working, compared to when neither of us were. Forty dollars compared to what Tuan and his friend could make or had access too. Those Lunar Fest meals cost less than a dollar."

"Maybe they were saving face though, because it was a fancy boat, proper etiquette is to each have a drink and a meal."

"So we were being rude." I nod.

"Though they were being egged on by the waiter. They had different expectations assuming we would pay."

"And they were so miserable after, especially Tuan."

"Remember, when we saw the boat and tried to talk them out of it. It looked too expensive for us."

"And we were in shorts and swimsuits. I remember feeling like an ugly blemish on a glimmering overly-glamourous stage."

We meet Tuan and Long in the evening but Tuan is still moody, angry we've left the hotel he chose for us, angry he has no money. Long is pleasant in comparison. He explains Tuan's background. He doesn't live with his family, but with his aunt and uncle. The boy and girl that I thought were brother and sister are cousins. His parents live outside the city on a farm. We learn from Long that the gap between living in a city and the lifestyle possible and living on a farm is immense. Tuan says little but I understand that with no money his Aunt will eventually have to send him back to his parents and his hopes for any kind of economic stability will decrease. The fan shop belongs to his aunt. He is studying computers but hasn't got enough money to pay. Of course, he wants our help. Long doesn't say this; he doesn't have to.

While Long talks, I try to ask Tuan for more details, but he is completely non-communicative. We leave them to walk up the street to our hotel. Tuan is not happy but offers to help us get food and take us to the bus depot before we leave the following night. We tell him we are fine, that we don't need his help, that he's done enough already, but he insists.

He knows which hotel we've moved to and says that with his help we will get better seats and a better price.

In the end, he shows up at the hotel early the next evening and asks us for the price of his tuition. In his mind we are the light in the tunnel, the gold at the end of the rainbow. When Tuan's realizes his hope of what we can do for him isn't going to pan out, his disappointment is bitter. The few dollars we might give will hardly help. His misery is a heavy weight between all of us.

Nonetheless, he escorts us to the bus depot. In the end, the conversation he had with his uncle does nothing for us. We are the last to be admitted onto the bus and there are no seats. Perched on bags of shoes wedged into the aisle, we settle for the long dark trip through the DMZ and into Laos.

I am walking past King's Pond near my house in Victoria and when I reach a certain curve in the trail (the scent, the ducks, the colour of the light) I am suddenly in Southeast Asia. Whatever I am remembering merges with the present moment as if two slides are pressed together, and then I'm back on the trail, in the real place again. Is it the writing of it that confuses my brain or is it that I'm still there? Vietnam is not a huge country. We were there from September 9–27; we had two months and three more countries ahead. Its impact on my memories is unrelenting. On the walk I am thinking about the Korean students I taught before we went to Japan. All the same age, we'd all go for drinks. Teacher and students, but we were also friends. Rupert and I visited them in Korea and they looked after us—showed us the city, took us to good restaurants, recommended a hotel. They felt responsible for me (us) because I had been their teacher. I think teacher trumped friends in many ways. It is naive of me to try to place us on equal terms. What do the anthropologists say about this kind of thing? All our cultural assumptions clouding reality.

Hua Hin, Thailand, October 27

After two days of rain we take most of what we own to the laundry down the street. Bliss. To wear clean clothes, clothes I've not washed by hand in cold water with my right thumb locking, bent. I wear an extra pair of shorts that has been buried in my bag for most of the trip, a bit snug for ridding and a bit short for around town. Since Hua Hin is touristy, with Germans and Americans in their beach-wear, I decide to wear them. The more well-dressed tourists are staying at the hotel with sculpted trees but at ours, anchored on stilts, the tide rises and falls under the floor boards of our room. When the rain briefly stops, we sit on the deck and eat. We wander the markets, umbrellas in hand, and then the rocky garbage-littered beach. We marvel, again, at the other travellers who've come by bus or train or moped or rented car. Their luxurious outfits, white jeans and ironed blouses. Teenagers behaving like regular teenagers and people speaking English in cafés where we go dumb, distracted by our foreign mother tongue. We pick up our clean laundry and carry it in plastic bags back to our room where we shake out our now dry and dusty panniers and repack.

You want to believe you rode away and their lives continued. While we wound our way south, Vietnam experienced the worst floods in a century. Who cares about misunderstandings when the waters come? Who cares about dictionaries and yellow mopeds when the water rises? In October and November more

than 650,000 homes were destroyed (not Yung's?). 793 people lost their lives (not Tuan?). Where were you when the first storm hit? From my journal: October 20 Chai Nat, 71km

"Today the landscape was ever changing. We seem to have left the huge fields behind and entered flood plains and swamps. Miles of flooded land, low lying mountains and bananas. There are bananas on vines, being roasted on grills, in bags, sweet and salty, crunchy, breaded, sold as chips. We crossed a flooded plain on a 1 bhat ferry—a car ferry no less—made from a large wooden raft. Large branches floated by. In the mist, back on the road, I saw the shape of Buddha, then I lost him. He sits out there ready to teach. His legs crossed and one hand draped, fingers relaxed and falling down his knee. Drops of rain."

All along you have been aware that your tickets mean release. Home. You knew, through talk and by the sight of flooded fields in Thailand, how bad the rains were. Is it only when popular tourist destinations, beaches and islands, are hit that it becomes world news. Or is it because you were so detached from the world that you didn't really know the damage until years later? You remember hearing of the floods in Vietnam and the faces of all those you'd met flashed past your eyes. Your maternal-like ownership of them. As if having met them you could cast some protective net around them. As you might your own children. Did they feel protective of us? Our Japanese friends did. We were like children. How this works, colonization. "You took me for a joke/ You took me for a child" (Alanis Morissette).

To Thalat near Keo Udon Lake on our way to Vang Vieng, Laos, October 6

"Uncle Freddy's for breakfast?" I ask my sleepy husband.

Vientiane has been good to us. Our hotel a calm haven with a giant, soft bed, a small window that looks out at the street, showers down the hall with almost-warm water and a western style toilet. I dress and turn on the television so we can pack to music—the same pop songs we've been hearing for the past two years—Cher's "Do You Believe in Life after Love" and the Backstreet Boys. These songs taunt and torture me down the roads of Asia. They are as pervasive as the sun and plantains. We finish packing, get our bikes out of storage and coast to the café.

Freddy is an ex-pat American with a Laotian wife. He hates and loves Laos. Having been part of the ex-pat community in Japan we have seen this before. Though we were there for only two years, anyone there for five or more formed a love-hate relationship with the country and its people. Freddy is no different. As we wait for our eggs and toast, I contemplate all the possible roads life can take. How we could have been Freddy in a few years, had we decided to stay in Japan. Happy to be away from Canada, yet missing it. Loving Japan, yet beginning to find fault with every aspect of its people and culture.

"Hey, Freddy," I holler, "we're heading to Vang Vieng, can you give us an idea how far it is." We'd been asking one of the Laos waiters, but her answer was vague at best. Freddy lumbers over full of mutters that are cut off by his raunchy smoker's cough.

"Don't ask the Laos," he says. "They have no concept of distance. They live here all their lives, travel up and down the highways of the country and yet can't tell you how far it is from one town to the next." He stands over us. Our copy of the *Lonely Planet* is open. We have been trying to calculate the distance from the tiny map provided. We want to know if we can get there in a day or if it will take two. If two, we want to know where we can stay tonight. Freddy is a good, though somewhat crotchety, resource.

"Ah, it's about a hundred kilometres, you guys can get there in a day."

"Is it pretty hilly?" Rupert asks. One hundred kilometres of flat road is an easy ride in a day. One hundred kilometres of constant climbing and dropping is next to impossible with a fully loaded bike after several days of rest. If it is hilly, we'd go sixty or eighty kilometers.

"Oh no, it's not bad. Gets mountainous further north of Vang Vieng. Great town, you'll love it."

We thank Freddy and after popping to the passport office to collect our passports and new Thai visas, we cycle north out of Vientiane. On the map, we are riding up a long dark line at the centre of the northern knuckle of the finger-shaped country, a finger that points south toward Cambodia, hooking around Thailand. I imagine that long dark line north as we ride up and down the winding hilly road. I imagine that we are climbing the side of the globe; that we are in the narrow passage of highway heading North, China on the next distant peak.

Bangkok and its modern bike shops are far south of us. This is a shame because Rupert's bike is falling apart. I can hear the seat post (with its ominous crack) squeak under his weight and mutter, "Why'd we trust the bike in the first place?" I ride behind, so I don't travel too far ahead, caught in my own thoughts, while Rupert has pulled over re-adjusting his axel. At this rate it will take an hour to cover five kilometres.

Finally, after a very slow twenty kilometres, we begin to make some progress. The road is beautifully paved and winds between farm land and clusters of houses. We come to a bridge with a sign in English and Laos, an Australian flag below. Developed countries have been helping Laos with road building, donating buses and other equipment for years. I assume Canada offers less aid than other countries, as the cost of our visas to Laos was almost twice what travellers from other countries have to pay. Perhaps Canada charges a reciprocal amount for Laos to get a Canadian Visa.

We stop at a road-side shelter for lunch. I love the country-side for the teak bus shelters that allow school children and farm workers a place to escape from the mid-day heat. Our bikes roll right into them or can lean against the stilt legs at the bottom. I take my shoes off and sit back, my head propped up against a post, protected under a green bandana, my hair sweaty underneath. Rupert gathers lunch things together. We have bread and potato chips and I crave a chip butty. Disgusting, I know, and less than nutritious, but this is all we have, and my body craves starch and salt, the crunch familiarity of chips. We will buy noodles and vegetables at the next town but for now it's a relief not having to worry how this meal will affect my blood sugars because as soon as we finish eating, we will burn it off. Our diet is the polar opposite of the Atkins' diet. We subsist almost totally on carbohydrates, with an egg or smattering of peanut butter thrown in now and again. Maybe tofu if we are lucky and cheese but only in more westernized towns. Vegetables if they are on offer. Fruit where we can find it. I've been vegetarian for years, Rupert a semi-vegetarian since we left Japan. He doesn't want to risk eating meat that has been hanging, cooked or uncooked, for days in the heat but will eat it to test for me and if he craves it. Most people don't worry about eating meat when they visit Asia but since I am a strict vegetarian anyway, Rupert decided to be cautious. Certainly I've had fewer stomach problems than he's had. Perhaps it hasn't been fair forcing him into the role of taste-tester, checking dishes to ensure they are "clean" for his paranoid veggie wife.

We also have banana chips bought at one of our many morning repair stops. As I crunch and crackle into my butty, Rupert nudges me and looks down the dirt road that meets the highway. A group of five school-girls approaches. Their smiles are huge and they can barely contain their excitement as they get closer. We ask them questions they don't understand but find incredibly funny. One finally gets brave enough to stroke the bleached hairs on my tanned arms. They all giggle. Rupert tries his usual stunts and hand games but for once the girls are more interested in me. One plops my helmet on her head. Yuck, I think to myself, that is one wet, smelly bike helmet. But she dances around while her friends giggle and point. Then she plops it on my head.

"Well, that's our cue, time to get going," Rupert says, saving me from other dress-up activities.

Being open minded seems a way to move away from colonialism. Did I think everyone in Asia was poor? Many Vietnamese had to relinquish great wealth to escape during and after the war. I remember so clearly a young girl in a café on our way to Vang Vieng. Her clothes and face were dust-covered. She was small and snotty nosed and sold something... little bags of dried banana chips and individual cigarettes. How would this girl manage if she were also diabetic? Her pretty lace shirt, her bare feet. Not so different, I think, from kids in their backyards here.

Scenes along the road: a ten-year-old girl holding her baby brother, his bare bottom nearly hitting the ground. We see no young women—all are babies, mothers, and grandmothers despite their age. The girl doesn't try to stop her brother's crying. She just bobs him in her small arms.

Vang Vieng, Laos, October 7

"Only one hundred kilometres, he said. No hills, he said." I am muttering again. Damn Freddy and his judgment of the Laos people. He didn't judge the distance between Vientiane and Vang Vieng any better, nor the contours of the road. I can't eat enough food on our second day going north. Between 12:30 and 2:30 I have eaten non-stop. Noodles, cycle, buns and peanut butter, cycle, yogurt drink, cycle, rice and eggs, cycle then, just before we reach town, I finish a PowerBar we'd started in the morning. An incredible amount of food that doesn't seem to satisfy my body's need. It is all the damned hills which we will have to ride again on our way back. I hate the idea of riding the same road twice, especially a road that constantly changes elevations.

"Freddy said it was a hundred kilometres to Vang Vieng but we've cycled... are you listening? We've cycled one hundred and ninety-three."

"No one understands distances when they are zooming off in a car," Rupert grumbles.

We are stressed about the ride back and our nearly expired visas. Just days ago I wanted nothing but cycling. Now I'm feeling the pressure of time and the need to hop on a bus for our return. Which, of course, is making me even crankier.

We coast into Vang Vieng, wondering as we approach each corner or curve in the road, if there will be a town there at all. We pass children bathing in irrigation pools, or small ponds off the river, it is hard to tell. *Sabai di. Sabai di. Sabai di falang!* The kids holler as we ride by. Then I blink, or the sun nestles behind a cloud, or someone resets the stage, and boom, we are in a bustling one-street touristy town.

Part of colonialism is judging the people through our own understanding of the world. Freddy's frustration with the Laotians and their lack of distance-knowledge. My frustration with Freddy because why would he know exactly how hilly a road is unless he had to ride it.

Remember: the cliffs and mountains of Vang Vieng, children, rice fields, bananas cooking on roadside grills, ten water buffalo, their heads poking out of a pond, loud moos and maws, barky chickens, monkeys, heavy rain showers, a walk under a tonne of mountain, Rupert and Mr. Keo singing folk and blues songs, my feet in red mud, voices loud and proud around us and the man following us from our guest house, offering to sell opium.

Tourists for a day, Vang Vieng, Laos, October 8
Rupert's Side of the Story

We joined a small tour group that consisted of a guide, Yvonne and me and two Dutch couples. We visited tribal villages, swam in a cave and floated down the Mekong River. It was an overcast windy day, but still in the thirties. We piled into a jeep and got dropped by a trail. The guide led us down a path along the edge of a field. Everyone kind of spread out as we walked. The guide and I fell back, walked side by side and talked about village life and history. He said that this village had helped the Americans during the American war in Vietnam and so after the war the tribes people were offered asylum in the US. The Americans feared there would be retribution. He said they sent money back from America so the village was doing better than many others. Then he fell into song. His voice sounded sad as he sang his folk song. Then I sang Greenland Fisheries and he sang another sad song as we came into the village. His voice rose over the landscape and filled the air and was carried off on the wind. We'd also been talking about kids, how five year olds looked after their two and three year old siblings. We saw a girl carrying her little brother on her back. She was barely older than he. We'd been talking about animals being used to attract tourists when we came to a shelter where monkeys were chained. One of the Dutch women paid to let the monkey sit on her back. Yvonne and I didn't get too close. We didn't want to support the business. It was such a little monkey with a funny red penis and a chain around his neck.

After the village we continued on to the caves. We followed a river bed down into a valley and then dropped into the cave. We had our bike lights and the guide had a candle, otherwise it was pitch dark but in we went. Albino spiders and the cool black water that we carefully slid into.

On the way back, we sang some more. I sang *Frère Jacque* and *Drunken Sailor* and the guide sang another sad Laos folk song. It felt like we were in a different country because we were doing a touristy thing. We got into inner tubes and floated back to Vang Vieng. For two hours we sat and watched the world go by until our legs were numb and cold. Then we guessed at our stop, swam to shore and pulled ourselves out. Back on the road, we had to figure out how to find the shop where we had left our backpack. There was something really freeing about knowing our accommodation was set for the night, because we were staying more than one night. Knowing our bikes and belongings were secure, we just walked and floated along. After showers we met the Dutch couples for garlic toast and French fries, called Fresh Friends on the menu. Because this was a tourist town, we felt as though we were in a community of foreigners, the way we'd felt in Japan. It was almost idyllic, like a holiday. Out on the bikes, we were on our own.

Rupert is in my studio with the photo album in his lap. Skinny girl, he says. I look funny in this picture, he says. Plasticky, I say. I like this one, he says, of a photo with him and a giant snake on his shoulders. That guide really didn't like the monkeys being chained, he says. We were so, so young, he says. We should make dinner, I say, rising to walk back to the house. We could have lettuce wraps from the garden lettuce. Let's order Thai food, he says. I pluck some weeds as I walk around the trampoline to get to the house. I watch him walk ahead of me. I hear his voice on the wind, the day so overcast and blustery that sounds seem as far off as memories.

We continue south on the main highway. The sun shines but we are battling excruciating wind. I need a break, so we stop; half an hour later I need another rest. The wind and hills wear me down, eat up my calories and strength. Millions of pineapples and coconut trees later, we ride down the streets of Bang Saphan. We have been here before, last year for New Year's. We came to Thailand from Japan and spent a week up north in Chiang Mai, did a mountain bike excursion for a few days, and then took a bus here. When we arrived at the bus depot, a man on a moped drove us and our two big backpacks to the Suan Luan resort.

Everything looks different now to eyes that have seen hundreds of miles of the country, hundreds of small towns. My feelings about this town—a town I perceived as small and isolated last year, when we couldn't easily get to it from our beach side resort —has changed. The road doesn't look remotely familiar as we turn off the main highway. We pass mini strip malls, auto shops, closed restaurants and cafes. Passing the Butterfly Café, I know in an instant that we have indeed arrived at a familiar place. We ride down a long hill, the very hill the two of us, our two packs and a driver drove down on the moped less than eleven months earlier. How different it looks. How much closer the town seems to the resort. How far I have come. How less afraid I am of the dark streets and hidden places of Thailand. How much more aware I am of what lies down those streets—often families, kind people and small cafés.

"There's the resort," I yell out, pedaling to catch up to Rupert.

The gravel driveway for the Suan Luan Resort is off to the left while the ocean is straight ahead. We enter and stop outside the open-air lounge and office. Behind this main building, small thatch-roofed huts sit in a half-circle with manicured grass between. The owner checks us into the same cabin as last time. The familiar hut has one room and a bathroom/shower. The roof is so slanted Rupert can only walk down the centre between front door and bathroom. We tuck our bikes under the overhanging roof and I get into my bathing suit, then lounge on a chair in the sun.

After a swim and a feast of the usual fried rice, we play scrabble in the main lounge. It all feels so familiar; I am delighted, relaxed. We can take a moment and not fret over the next one.

Soaked in sunscreen that drips with sweat off the tip of my nose, glides down my sunglasses, I've pedaled until my bottom is scaled, my legs rose-coloured muscles. The thumb on my right hand locks due to the miles of holding my handlebars and the days of washing socks. By this point I ride in my sandals. I've sung every song I know to myself, to the air and trees, to my husband. I've relived moments of my past, dreamt the many possible futures. The sun stings my eyes, eyes fixed on the white line that divides me from fast moving trucks. Eyes that saunter into the bushes, see shapes that are not there: lizards in shards of coconut, snakes in blown tires, a snorting buffalo off in the shadows in a pile or red dirt, its eyes, unblinking shards of glass.

Tanah Rata, Cameron Highlands, Malaysia, November 24

After a night of vomiting and diarrhea, Rupert sits on the edge of my hospital bed. I desperately want to leave and get back on the road. Our time is pinching up at the end of this road. For so long it has snaked ahead of us but suddenly we can see the mouth.

"If we bus back to Tuluk Intan tomorrow," Rupert says, trying to gain my attention, "there's no way we can ride all the way to Kuala Lumpur and still see the city before our flight on Saturday."

Tomorrow is Tuesday. A day ago I lost all the liquid in my system; I am weak and shaky. We sit in silence until the doctor comes in to take my pulse and temperature.

"How you feel?" he asks, pumping the arm band as he talks.

"Much better," I say. "Can I leave today? What was wrong with me?"

"You have no parasites," he says, "It is the rainy weather, brings out the viruses. Yes, you can go. Your blood pressure is very low, very low." He sucks his breath and shakes his head, but releases me.

The fact that I have no parasites concerns me. No parasites means that the vomiting and diarrhea could be due to my blood sugars. I could be on the border of ketoacidosis or prolonged high blood sugars.

We wait for a nurse to come and remove the IV, then head downstairs to fill my prescription and pay for two days in hospital.

"So, five ringgit for the medicine and hospital stay," says the young man behind the counter. He hands me no medicine, just rehydration crystals to add to my drinking water to replace lost salts and nutrients. The total cost of hospitalization comes to about a dollar fifty.

"Only five?" I say, looking him in the eyes.

The man smiles and hands over a paper bag of individually wrapped doses of drinking crystals, careful to touch my hand slightly. "You be careful now."

Rupert and I walk down the now familiar, incredibly short main street. We stop at a grocery store for some juice and snacks. I am in no mood to eat but Rupert is starving so we stop at the Indian restaurant we ate at on our first day. I test my blood and nibble on a few things, my head and heart heavy.

"We'll have to bus all the way to KL," I say so quietly Rupert barely hears me. He doesn't answer, simply nods, his eyes on me. "There's no point in missing out on the culture of the city," I add.

When was the last time we cycled, I wonder? Was that all a dream? Do we really have bikes waiting for us at the bottom of this mountain? Aren't we in a different world now? In five days, we'll be in another ghostly familiar alien world—home.

Four times a day I puncture my skin with a small needle. Four to six times a day, I prick a finger and bleed onto a small stick to measure my blood sugar levels and adjust my insulin doses. I eat breakfast, snack, lunch, snack, supper, snack. I do these things so I can live. Having diabetes balances me on a bicycle, the sun in my face, my feet spinning. I could fall to one side or the other. I could just keep pedaling. My eyes looking to the long and distant horizon. My body balanced on this machine is a courtship with gravity; the balance of food and insulin and activity is a courtship with life. What can I do each day but choose the way I live? We choose, so we perch and pedal. Or we choose caution and speed over desire and expectation. We let the experiences we have

created fill and inform us. We go in with great expectations and come out with immeasurable experiences.

"You can't do everything," my dad always tells me.

We cycled 3719 kms of a 4568 km distance. The 850 kms we bussed does not negate the cycling. I have to tell myself this. I have to remind myself that nothing vanishes, not the euphoria of cycling nor the passion for each curve and bump in the road. I have to remind myself that it all matters, it all counts: every dog that followed or chased us, every child who waved or adult who gave what we needed, who smiled or bowed or showed us how to live in this part of the world, where we do not always know our place or who we are.

To be sick. To be overly emotional. To be ashamed. To be noticed. To stand out. To not stand out. To be in the spotlight. To sit in the dark corner. To be forgotten. To go unnoticed. To be petted and stroked. To be scowled at. To smile. To forget the root of the self. To be ashamed. To draw the bear's eye. To draw the snake's. To not draw it. To ask for help. To not ask for help. To refuse. To refuse an ending. To refuse to hope. To stand out in a crowd. To mark the land. To leave no mark. To be marked. By the land. By the people.

In the middle of the night the bus lurches crossing the DMZ. It's dark. Two white women board the bus. Nicki and Julie. Young nurses from England. We ride to Savannakhet chatting the whole way.

To cross the Thai-Lao Friendship Bridge into Thailand we have to take a bus that does not want us. We have to take the bus because in Laos we ride on the right and in Thailand we will ride on the left. It is a short bridge but we may not ride across it. When we finally get across and are ready to go, the first things I see is an Elephant Taxi. I wonder if he has walked over the bridge and how confusing that must be for the elephant.

Rupert reads the Bible. I read whatever I can find. In Udon Thani I buy *Touch the Dragon* by Karen Connelly. A book about a young woman's experience as a Rotary Exchange student in Thailand.

I fear that what is written here leaves too much out. Taking shelter in a rubber tree forest and being invited to the manor house for tea. The Wat surrounded by rice fields, its glistening gold trim. Laughter. The many, many days in a row when I was strong, not ill, healthy, at my best.

I fool around and I fall into the ocean off Malaysia onto a sea anemone. Poor creature, but even worse, my hand swells. If anyone falls, it is me.

Murtabaka. Chai Tea. Popcorn from Tiger gas stations. Spring rolls from Danang that I can still sometimes taste. Scents along the road—the bad ones, like garbage trucks and durian fruit. But also, spices, papayas, bananas, elephants' dusted skin, clean sheets, just showered skin, bike grease, road dust, damp cement, grass.

Rupert's yellow cycling shirt. The mantis he can't get off it. The Louise Guest House, my sister's name offering a home.

I am running out of pages. I have left so much out. I fear that when I finish all the rich memories will be cemented into this version. Where am I now? I am at my desk. It is mid-summer. Years have passed but I remember the smiling faces, the feeling of being a minority, the frustration and the desire to connect. I am the other on her bicycle in a far off place. I am here and there at once. Does anyone care about two young people riding bicycles in far off countries not for control or gain but just curiosity? The world is full of people who are the same and different at once. Am I witnessing something? Witness to my own distant and present story.

"Rupert," I whisper and squeeze his arm.

Three hours ago we caught the early bus down the mountain, picked up our bikes and boarded a bus for Kuala Lumpur. Now we are on the outskirts of the city. Highway overpasses by the millions are strung together and converge as the bus rumbles up and over one pass, then exits and goes up and over, then down and around the next. I feel like we are caught in a cat's cradle but the driver seems to know what he is doing. We haven't passed through many towns on the way here and we haven't stopped once. I have watched the road the whole way.

Rupert opens his eyes. "Are we almost there?"

The city streets sprawl out all around going up and down, the closer to the centre we get the narrower the lanes, the more chaotic the traffic.

"Kuala Lumpur," yells the bus driver and we gather our things. My heart is in my throat. Excitement?

"We have bikes," Rupert informs the driver, who puts the bus into park and follows us outside. Our bikes are in the storage compartment under the bus.

The minute we step off, the heat hits us. In seconds I am soaked and shaking. After a week of cool Cameron Highlands' temperatures and a day on an air conditioned bus, the sudden heat shocks the system.

"Aha, you see, we will have to ride again," Rupert says consulting our map. We are miles out of the main part of the city. We negotiate our bags onto bikes and I feel a sense of déjà vu flood over me. Of course, I've done this before and not so long ago. The week in the mountains feels like a year on a distant planet. My legs wobble as we push off from the bus centre just as they did that first day.

Despite the shakes and the doubts, I feel a growing sense of excitement as we settle into our ride, as we approach a new place, a place about which I am curious but know little. A huge city with a fascinating history and clusters of cultures.

We don't get far before I need some juice and a second to catch my breath. Once I stabilize, we are off again, two cyclists surrounded on all sides by utter chaos—mosques, colourful Hindu temples and Catholic churches. The twin towers of this busy city point to the sky in the distance and the noise and chaos of Little India streams around us like the silk shawls of a sari. Rupert stays close as we cycle past huge, coiling incense sticks and enter Chinatown.

"Too far," Rupert stops and looks back. "We've overshot."

Back and back we go until we stumble onto a busy intersection off a main street with one, two, three guest houses. I lean with the bikes, while Rupert hoofs up a set of stairs. The familiar and final time, I think, fleetingly as minutes later we heave our bikes in after us. The Backpackers Traveller's Lodge, our last stop, last home away from home.

Am I moving forward or backward through time? Am I bus-antsy in Laos because I know how this will end? I don't feel disappointed, I feel elated (light headed, low blood pressure?). Here I am ready to go home. I am ready to ride. Here I am drawn closer to the Buddha on the distant hill. Here, antsy to find a toilet, some food, some shade, a smile. Here I am. I can smell the incense. I can feel that tired. I am there. I am here.

Leaving Hanoi, Vietnam, September 12

We head back into the chaos of traffic toward the train tracks, following them south out of the city along the main national highway. We pass Vietnamese women carrying baskets of bread or vegetables, even bricks balanced on their heads. We pass old French Colonial two-story houses with peaked red roofs and white-washed brick walls. Most are in varying degrees of decay. The frame of walls in some of the houses are intact but few are perfectly formed. They remind me of Greek statues that are missing arms, legs and faces. One house reveals its bones, layers of bricks that should be covered with an outer coating of stucco. Dusty piles lie at the house's feet like shed skin. Some houses are missing doors. Shocking holes pock outer walls as if hit by a bomb. Dampness or decay, I wonder, or war?

We begin to forgo the rules of right of way. Instead, give way to anything larger and faster, even a dog or water buffalo. All along the road, as it changes from busy city street to narrower single lane, we attract attention. The road and the people on it take a deep breath to watch us pass. We share the road with few cars or trucks, more mopeds, even more bicycles, like the woman delivering still-live chickens which hang from their tied feet off her handlebars. She wears Aoi-Dai, Vietnam's traditional clothing of white pants and a long white Chinese-collared shirt. She waves as she passes and her companions, one with two huge baskets filled with greens, another with long bamboo poles balanced on handlebars, and a third carrying baskets of vegetables, all smile broadly as they pass, their quiet laughter echoing above the sounds of traffic.

I am on my bike. I am riding fast through Cedar Hill Golf course to get home to switch to my car to pick my son up from school. It is early in the year, but it is warm. Climate change, I think, as I speed past the ducks in their toxic pond. My sugars are dropping and I will have to text a friend to get my son because I'm not going to make it. I am in my studio. I am on my back in my mother's garden. I am small. I am so small some days it feels like everything penetrates my thin white skin. In 1999 I cycled in Southeast Asia with my husband. Some days I am still there. On my bike. In another country. The roads have etched themselves into the skin of my belly. The sun has marked my freckles. In 2001 9/11. In 2004 a Tsunami destroyed a jetty I ride my bike on in Malaysia. Nothing remains. I could not retrace the path we took. The roads are imagined. There was no google maps. We did not mark the landscape. Today I follow a path along the ocean, passing the shipping yards of my city. I pause at a street crossing, as the sun is briefly covered by cloud. The road is wet from days of rain, the air warm, humid enough that I am on another road, on my bike, again.

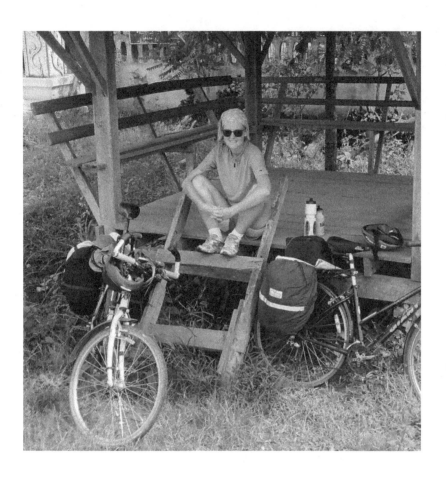

Chart of days and distances

DAY	DATE	PLACE	DISTANCE/ NOTES
1	0908	leave Japan for Taiwan	
2	0909	arrive Hanoi	40km
3	0910	in Hanoi	15km
4	0911	in Hanoi	
5	0912	to Phu Ly	59km
6	0913	to Pho Len	88km
7	0914	to Cang	67km
		bus to 15km north of Vinh	
		cycled to Cua Lo	15km
8	0915	Rest day Vinh	16km
9	0916	to Ha Tinh	76km
10	0917	Ky M... (near Ngang Pass	80km
11	0918	to Dong Hoi	78km
12	0919	Dong Hoi to Dong Ha	99km
13	0920	to Hue	66km
14	0921	around Hue	30km
15 - 17	0922-24	in Hue to Danang and Hoi An	
18	0925	Danang—China Beach	
19	0926		
20	0927	on bus to Savannakhet	
21	0928	in Savannakhet	
22	0929	in Savannakhet	
23	0930	to Tha Khek—bus	
24	1001	rode, by car to Pakkading River,	
		rode to Paksan 30km/ 128km (car)	42 km
25	1002	to Wat Phra Bat Phonsavan	
		bus to Vientianne	73 km
26	1003	Vientianne	
27	1004	Vientianne	
28	1005	to Buddha Park and back	48km

29	1006	in Thalat near Keo Udon Lake	90km	
30	1007	Vang Vieng	103km	
31	1008	in Vang Vieng		
32	1009	Vang Vieng		
33	1010	bus back to Vientianne		
		cycled to Nong Khai	20+km	
		crossed Thai-Laos Friendship bridge,		
		cycled to Nong Khai		
34	1011	Udon Thani	61.35km	
		to town	54km	
35	1012	to Naklang	83 km	
36	1013	to Nong Hin	88km	
37	1014	to Lom Kao—straight up	81km	eye infection
38	1015	Lom Sak—rest day	13 km	
39	1016	bus and cycled to small town		
		bus	50km	
		ride	43 km	
40	1017	Phitsanulok	51km	
41	1018	Pratchit	70km	
42	1019	Nakhon Sawan	121 km	prov. capital
43	1020	Chai Nat	71km	
44	1021	Bangkok		
45	1022	Bangkok		
46	1023	Bangkok		
47	1024	Nakhon Pathon	56km	
48	1025	Hua Hin, riding and busing—the rain		
49	1026	Hua Hin		
50	1027	Prechup Khiri Khan	102km	
51	1028	Bang Saphan (Suan Luan Resort)	102 km	
52	1029	guest house by beach	63 km	
53	1030	Lang Suan	116 km	

54	1031	Phun Phin	97 km
		hitched last	30km
55	1101	Surat Thani	12km rest day
56	1102	Thung Song	145.1 km
57	1103	Phattalung	91 km
58	1104	Hat Yai	90km
59	1105	rest day, bussed to Songlkla in eve.	
60	1106	to Changklang	80km
		to border	70 km
		to first town in Malaysia	10km
61	1107	Alor Setar	70km
62	1108	to Penang, George Town	100km
63	1109	in George Town	
64	1110	Ferenghi (beach town on Penang)	12km
65	1111	beach	
66	1112	beach	
67	1113	Pinang—Taiping	95 km
68	1114	P. Pangkhor	114km island
69	1115		
70	1116	Sitiawan	23km
71	1117	Tuluk Intan	59km
72	1118	Tanah Rata—bus	bikes left in Tuluk Intan
73	1119	Tanah Rata—Cameron Highlands	bus
74	1120	Tanah Rata	
75-78	1121-24		
79	1125	Kuala Lumpur	bus
80	1126		
81	1127	fly home	
82	1128	arrive in Vancouver	
		TOTAL	3719 km

Notes to sections

I have used anglicized spellings of village and town names throughout. Though I carefully noted places in my journal, small villages have been impossible to find again on maps or Google to verify. So much has changed. Any errors are mine.

On page 41 quote from *By-Line: Selected Articles and Dispatches of Four Decades* by Ernest Hemingway, edited by William White, 1998, Scribner. I also quote from *Journey Not The Arrival Matters: An Autobiography Of The Years 1939 to 1969* by Leonard Woolf, 1989, Mariner Books.

Throughout I quote lyrics from Alanis Morisette's album *Jagged Little Pill*. On page 11 from "Right Through You," pages 177–178 "That I would be Good," page 198 "All really want," and page 215 "Right Through You."

On page 39 I quote from the movie *Steel Magnolias*, 1989, Herbert Ross director.

On page 46 I quote my specialist Dr. David Miller from his written notes.

On pages 51 and 58 I quote from a personal interview with Maria Lahiffe.

On page 60 I quote from *A Tale for the Time Being*, Ruth Ozeki, 2013, Viking.

On page 67 I quote from *Global Car, Motorcycle,* and *Bike Ownership* in "1 info-graphic" by Tanvi Misra from *The Atlantics' City Lab Magazine*, April 17, 2015. On pages 71 and 142 I quote from *A Philosophy of Boredom* by Lars Svendsen, 2004, Reaktion Books Ltd.

On page 74 Rupert sings the theme song to *Gilligan's Island*, which ran from 1964–1967 and forever after as reruns. Produced by United Artists Television.

On pages 77 and 106 I quote from *The Other* by Ryszard Kapuściński.

On pages 84 and 186 I quote from *Ru* by Kim Thúy, translated by Sheila Fischman, 2012, Vintage Canada.

On page 91 I mention Little Bee by Chris Cleave, 2008, Sceptre, UK.

On page 94 I quote from *The Inconvenient Indian* by Thomas King, 2012, Anchor Canada.

On pages 97–98 I quote from Steven Heighton's chapbook *Paper Lanterns*, 2006, Palimpsest Press.

On pages 134–135 I quote William Hazlitt, from his essay "On the feeling of immortality in youth" internet archive.

On page 154 I pull a quote from *The Globe and Mail*, Globe Focus, "Whitewashed: The Real Reason Donald Trump got elected" by Doug Saunders, Saturday November 12, 2016

On pages 161-162 I talk about the movie *The Thomas Crown Affair*, 1999, John McTiernan, director.

On page 171 I quote Cheryl Strayed's *Wild*, 2012, Knopf and the movie *Wild* 2014, directed by Jean-Marc Vallée.

On page 180 I quote *The Wheels of Chance* by H.G. Wells, 1896, J.M. Dent & Co.

On page 191 I quote from Kathleen Winter's *Boundless*, 2014, House of Anansi.

On page 203 I quote the lines "Danang me, Danang me, why don't they get a rope and hang me" from the movie *Good Morning Vietnam*, 1987, directed by Barry Levinson.

In small towns I hear the music from *The Good, the Bad and the Ugly*, 1966, Sergio Leone, director and music composed by Ennio Morricone.

Throughout we quote song lyrics from Cher's "Do You Believe in Life after Love" and The BackStreet Boys "Tell me Why," these songs followed us everywhere along with "La Isla Bonita" by Madona.

We are guided through this journey with the help of *South-East Asia on a Shoestring*, 10th edition, 1999, Lonely Planet Publications Pty Ltd.

Acknowledgements and thanks

Rupert and I cycled in Southeast Asia in 1999, returning home at the end of the millennium surrounded by talk of what would happen when the clocks swung to 2000. Nothing much did though we suffered terrible reverse culture shock and had to find jobs and a place to live. I published a few pieces on cycling in Victoria's *Times Colonist*, one on Vietnam, twenty-five years after the war and another on bicycles in Japan. Shortly afterwards, in 2001, I started writing a weekly cycling column for the TC called *Spoke 'n' Word* which ran until the summer of 2004 when we moved to the UK for a year. In 2002 I returned to the University of Victoria to continue my Writing degree. I wrote poems and parables with Derk Wynand and creative nonfiction with Lynne van Luven. They both allowed me to do directed studies. A huge thank you to Lynne van Luven for her encouragement as I wrote the first draft of *Sugar Ride*. Excerpts of this memoir appeared early on in *Monday Magazine* and *Diabetes Dialogue*. Rupert and I gave presentations to cycling coalitions in Victoria and on Salt Spring Island and I also gave a presentation to the Juvenile Diabetes Association AGM. Most recently, I recited "The Longest Day" at the Belfry in the spring of 2016 as part of *The Flame* with thanks to Deborah Williams.

After my work with Lynne, I left the manuscript behind and got swept up in poetry for several years beginning with my MA in Creative Writing: Poetry at the University of East Anglia in 2004.

In 2012 the poems inspired by this trip were published in a limited edition chapbook with JackPine press titled *Bicycle Brand Journey* with accompanying Blake-like art by Regan Rasmussen. The poems and art co-exist on large hand-made playing cards as if Rupert and I were playing cribbage in a quiet guesthouse somewhere just off the road. Thanks to Regan Rasmussen for her artistic eye and friendship.

When the poetry book came out, I was drawn back into those long days of cycling. I worked with Betsy Warland and we discussed the key predicament in the manuscript and explored the liminal spaces in travel. Huge thanks to Betsy for her imaginative questions and her awesome guidance. I'm so grateful for her insight and friendship. In the final stages I worked with Patricia Young, who chewed through my sentences marking them with "??" and sometimes phoned me with encouragement. Huge thanks Patricia for her questions that led to clarifications and her awesomeness. Finally, thanks to Carmine Starnino who moved things around, asked for more, and edited for sense and style. Thank you so much to all of these writers and editors. Thanks also to my specialist Dr. David Miller who read through flagged pages and asked questions like—"what was your back up plan?" and to Aimee Parent Dunn and Dawn Kresan at Palimpsest, they have ventured into new territory with me here and have been amazing as ever to work with.

Editors are essential but so are the people who encourage you to go in the first place, or at least don't discourage. Thanks Tamar Thompson my beloved friend who was planning a trip to Thailand in the spring of 1999 and let me join her. Thank you Midori and Masanobu Karashima, our family in Nogata, Japan. We left everything we owned with the Karashimas when we left Japan with only our bicycles. Thanks also to the Okabe family for housing us our last days in Japan and driving us and our bikes to the airport. Thanks to Vi Nguyen and Jim Solomita, also members of the JET programme, whom we met up with in Hanoi for our first few days. Vi and her family left Vietnam during the war and Vi's dad kindly wrote us a letter in Vietnamese explaining all the drugs and needles we carried. Thanks also to the people we met along the way who offered snacks, conversation, challenged us or laughed with us, especially the children for their curiosity and courage in approaching us to say hi.

I must also thank friends with whom I've had deep conversations on wealth and poverty, skin colour, money, health, thresholds, quantum physics and colonialism. We have explored how screwed up the world is and how important it is to keep asking the questions and making it better. Thanks Terry Ann Carter, Barbara Pelman, Anita Lahey, John Barton, Cynthia Woodman Kerkham who gave this book its name, and Maria Lahiffe who is quoted in the book for her experiences in Ghana. Thanks Rhonda Ganz designer and friend for our editing weekend away, Nancy Yakimosky for photographs and Planet Earth Poetry for years of great poetry and fellowship.

And finally, my family. I thank my parents Rita and Clive Blomer for passing on their curiosity and adventurous spirit and for managing to meet all those years ago in Africa. Thanks to my father-in-law Robert Gadd for his many stories and my mother-in-law Sara Gadd who is not with us anymore but would have read this in one sitting. I thank my sister for bringing PowerBars to Japan, where, jet-lagged, we made her start a cycling holiday and for teasing me when we were kids until I figured out how to balance on a bike! Thanks to my beautiful son Colwyn for understanding that mom writes. We will take him to Asia someday soon and maybe inspire or offer refuge to a young couple on bicycles.

And finally, Rupert: thanks for being cyclist, co-conspirator in this adventure, husband and friend. Thanks for the questions and clarifications and thanks for being interviewed for your "parts" in the book. Thanks also for your sense of humour, your determination, your care when I was unwell, your mechanical skills with bikes, your knowledge of diabetes in a pinch, and our many years of marriage, laughter and adventures. In 2017 we will be married twenty years, yet I can still smell the dirt and durian fruit, can hear our tread on the road and see you just ahead of me encouraging a dog to chase so you can squirt it in the face from your water bottle.

If I am in a photo, Rupert took it, otherwise I did.

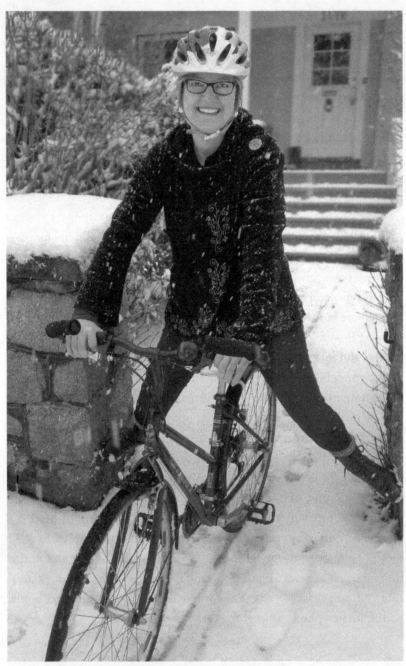
Author photo by RUPERT GADD

Author Biography

Yvonne Blomer is the Poet Laureate of Victoria, British Columbia. Born in Zimbabwe, she has lived in Japan and England and has cycled in Southeast Asia, Japan, Mexico, Canada, France and the UK. Her most recent poetry collection is *As if a Raven* (Palimpsest Press, 2014). Her first book of poems a broken mirror, fallen leaf was shortlisted for the Gerald Lampert Memorial Award. Blomer is the past Artistic Director of Planet Earth Poetry and co-edited the anthology *Poems from Planet Earth* (Leaf Press, 2013). She is also the editor of the anthology *The Pacific Ocean: Protecting our Endangered Coast* (Caitlin Press, 2017). Yvonne resides in Victoria, BC. www.yvonneblomer.com.